MASSAGE

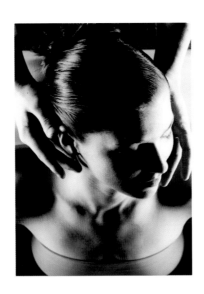

an introduction to
MASSAGE

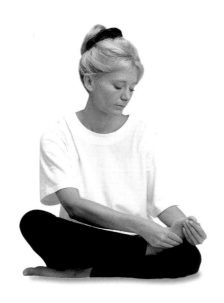

Vivienne Simberg

p

This is a Parragon book
This edition published in 2005

Parragon
Queen Street House
4 Queen Street
Bath BA1 1HE, UK

Copyright © Parragon 2002

This book was created by
THE BRIDGEWATER BOOK COMPANY

Photography Ian Parsons

A CIP catalogue record for this book is
available from the British Library

ISBN 1-40544-619-6

Printed in Indonesia

Contents

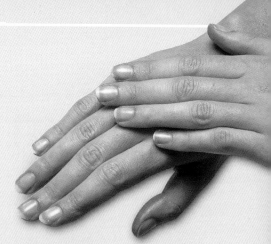

The Origins and History of **Massage**

Massage is a safe and effective combination of techniques that almost anyone can learn. It is a holistic therapy and offers benefits for the physical, mental, spiritual and emotional wellbeing of the person giving the massage as well as the person receiving it. It works well on young and old, male and female, and can even be applied as a self-help therapy.

Massage has been practised medicinally and therapeutically in the streets, homes, workplace and in hospitals for centuries, from the earliest civilisations to the present day. Cave paintings and art from Ancient Egyptians depict the use of oils and touch for purifying, healing and beautifying body and soul. Gladiators and soldiers were massaged before battle to promote fitness, and after battle to aid recovery. The Phoenicians and the Greeks record massage as early as 450BCE, and there are studies by Hippocrates on the use of massage in

Massage has played its part in many traditions and religions from around the world for centuries.

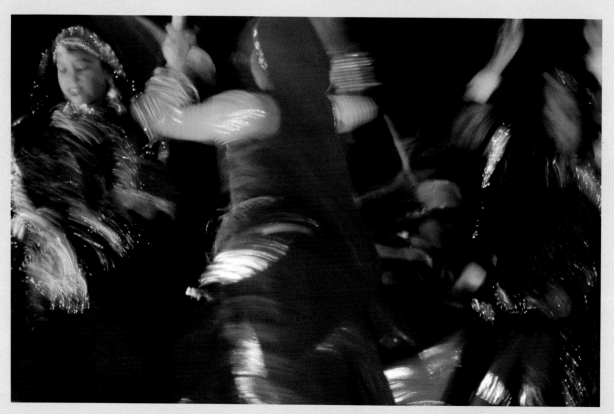

the early days of medicine. Biblical records tell us of the power of touch-healing from Jesus and the Hebrews. In the Roman era, Cleopatra records receiving massage; books dating back to the Crusades in the Middle Ages have been found that record massage; and massage was even used during the First World War to relax the wounded in the absence of medical supplies.

If you have never really given any thought to massage, think again.

Through touch, massage plays a vital part in the healing process. It improves physical health and general well-being, as well as clarity and function of the mind, enabling you to reach your spiritual side. Touch is appreciated by all, especially those who rarely have any physical contact in their everyday lives, such as the elderly or infirm. Massage is truly a gift of touch.

The word massage derives from the Latin word *mass* and the Arabic word *massa*, meaning to rub or press gently. It is a comforting hold when you feel unwell – most of us can recall the feeling of well-being when mum or dad rubbed their magic hands on our bumps, bruises and scratches, or placed a cool hand on a fevered brow to see if we had a temperature. When you have a headache, you will instinctively place the palm of your hand across your brow and rub gently. When you have received bad news, it is good to have a friend's shoulder to lean on and to receive a comforting cuddle and hug, or to have your shoulder rubbed in a reassuring manner or a gentle

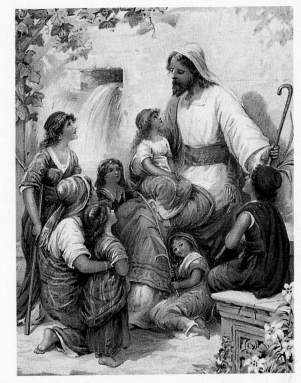

The power of a healing touch – the so-called laying-on of hands – is known in many religions, including Christianity.

squeeze applied to your arm. We have all at some time received massage in some form.

Therapeutic massage is a structured extension of this instinctive touching. It is not one technique but many that can be used alone or in combination. Where illness or discomfort is caused by problems with muscle or joints, where there is problem with circulation or with the lymphatic system, or when something is causing a blockage in energy flows, massage will be able to help. But it is also useful for emotional or psychological problems, where what is needed is a boost to confidence or to self-esteem.

We instinctively seek the soothing touch of those who care for us when we are in pain.

Massage in Everyday Life

Massage comprises many techniques and a therapist may be able to offer one or more in isolation or combination. But you don't need to go to a therapist to appreciate some of the more fundamental aspects of massage that are probably already part of your everyday life.

When you have a busy day and schedule ahead, you are perhaps more likely to take a shower than a bath. You use a towel to dry yourself, using a vigorous scrubbing motion, and as you scratch and rub from side to side you stimulate the blood flow ready for action.

If you relax in a warm bath and add aroma, candlelight and soft music, you will feel more inclined to caress your skin gently with a soapy mitt with smooth long strokes. As you feel more and more relaxed, repeat the strokes softly and make them longer, from your shoulder to your fingertips.

When you dry yourself, you will tend to be more gentle, wrapping the towel around you as you lay on your bed for a while meditating or perhaps contemplating what you are going to wear for a forthcoming occasion.

Massage can be applied in daily life in caring for yourself and others. Following an injury, you might apply a compress to the affected area, adding a licensed brand-name antiseptic to a bowl of water, or using water on its own. Dip a cotton pad in the water, squeeze it out and massage the area gently, avoiding direct contact with any broken skin. Work gently around the injured site and massage towards your heart to stimulate blood supply and lymphatic drainage.

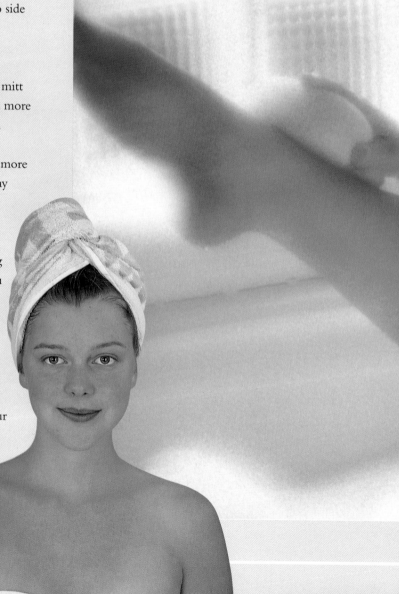

A good long soak in a bath is a form of massage known as hydrotherapy, and can soothe and calm or invigorate as needed.

Apply a cold compress when heat is present around the injury, but apply a hot compress if the injury is muscular and the affected area is cold. Alternating hot and cold compresses helps to reduce swelling in the damaged tissues.

How often do you sit in stockinged or bare feet on your bed or your couch, holding your feet as you watch the television?

You are doing yourself more good than you realise, as the study of reflexology confirms that anatomically the feet map the pattern of the body's internal organs and structure. Each bump and contour tells you how your body has worn and how efficiently you are operating internally.

Rubbing your feet after day of standing is a form of self-massage that is done instinctively.

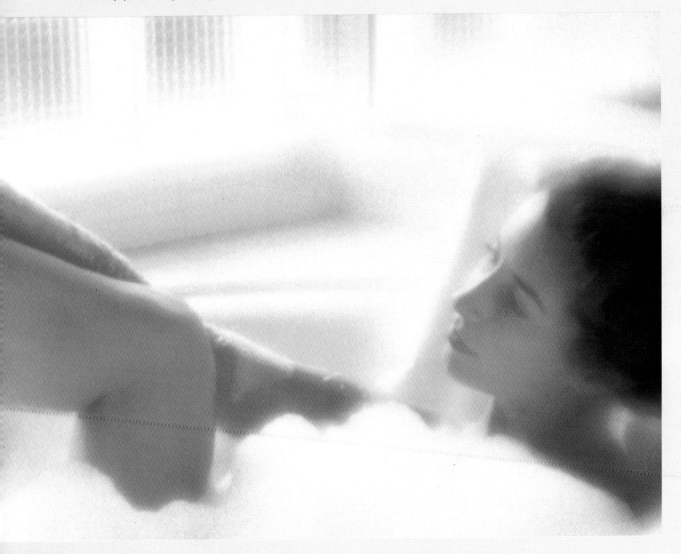

Who is Massage **Suitable** for?

Massage is suitable for all living, feeling, sentient beings – not just for the ill or infirm. We can all benefit greatly from the caring touch of another person.

Massaging babies helps with the development of their motor movement and coordination – and massage can help parents, too. All parents need regular breaks from busy schedules, and they will benefit greatly from making time for themselves. The feeling of well-being that massage brings will help them to cope with the worry of taking care of a child, as well as releasing some of the stress and strain that parenthood can cause at home and at work. A happy, relaxed parent is generally more fun to be with, and can continue refreshed to contribute to the well-being of all the family members, or meet heavily demanding schedules at work.

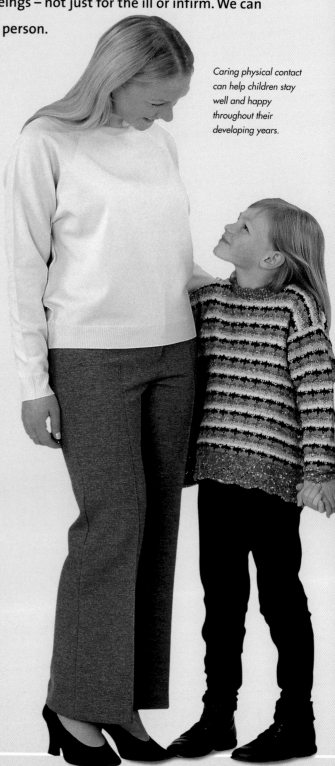

Caring physical contact can help children stay well and happy throughout their developing years.

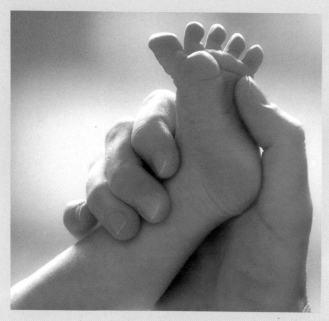

There has been a resurgence of interest in the benefits that baby massage can bring to both carer and child.

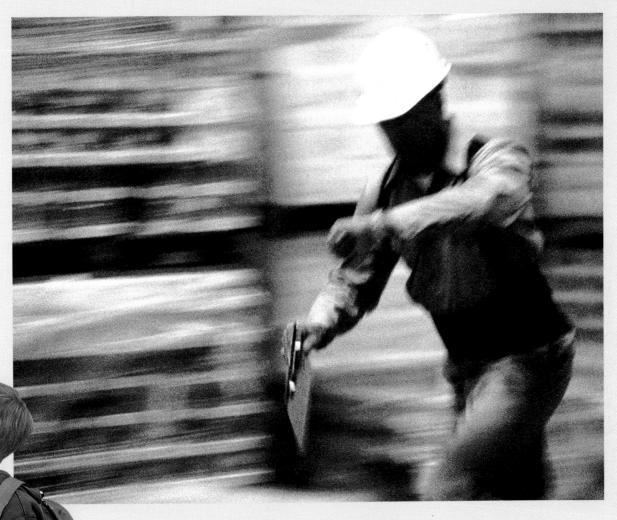

Children experience stress caused by the pressures of their academic and social environments, as well as trying to live up to family expectations. Massage can help relieve and reduce anxiety in young people and reduce unsociable behaviour patterns in adolescent years. Massage also helps to alleviate growing pains and minor injuries.

Older people will also benefit physically and psychologically from massage, which assists and often improves circulation, and reduces the risk of muscle strain. These factors allow the elderly to continue following an active lifestyle.

The pressures of daily life take their toll. The compulsion to work long hours subjects

It is important to take time out to relax if stress is not to lead to serious illness. Massage can be an important element of relaxation.

the body to pressures that it will not be able to cope with without some programme of maintenance. The temptation is to think that if nothing hurts then everything is all right. However, constant stress builds up tension in the body until eventually something has to give.

Whether stress manifests itself as aches and pains in the muscles and joints or as mental dis-ease, massage can help alleviate it, by restoring balance and releasing energy blockages. In some illnesses and conditions, however, massage should be avoided. These are outlined in the precautions section on the following pages.

PRECAUTIONS

Avoid massage in the following conditions, instances and disorders:

DURING THE FIRST THREE MONTHS OF PREGNANCY (see opposite) .

DURING MENSTRUATION, as massage can make the blood flow heavier.

DIABETES – the severity of diabetes levels vary, but when the condition is severe the patient can be unable to detect pain.

HEART CONDITIONS – with conditions diagnosed, or when angina is suspected, avoid massage due to the increase in venous flow. Varying blood pressure brought on by increased heart rate could induce shock.

VARICOSE VEINS, or history of thrombosis. Do not massage over broken or varicose veins as the blood supply is impaired in this area. Massage will increase blood flow and flood the over-worked capillaries and veins, possibly causing coagulation and affecting blood flow to the heart. Professionally trained therapists may effleurage gently when advised by consultant or general practitioner of patient.

ARTHRITIS – massage produces excess heat in the inflammatory stage. Gentle stroking in the sequential stage is permitted, however.

RECENT SCAR-TISSUE SITES, whether scarring is the result of accident or surgery – avoid the localised site as skin and body tissues are still repairing for up to six months (and up to two years for major surgical sites).

INCREASED BODY TEMPERATURE, as massage could spread an infection.

INFLAMMATION, as this could be due to fatty deposits causing a cyst, and massage will spread the infection. Inflammation is also the body's way of protecting the damaged area beneath.

SEVERE SKIN PROBLEMS, such as eczema or psoriasis – massage can add to dermal irritation.

OPEN WOUNDS, CUTS AND BRUISING – apply only light touch drainage massage around the site, to assist the blood flow toward the heart and encourage healing where bruising is present. Oil may aggravate an open wound.

INJURIES TO MUSCLES AND JOINTS – these are best left to a professional therapist.

WHEN UNDER TREATMENT from another practitioner, seek permission from that professional as natural plant-derived chemical properties are found in some oils that will contraindicate or counteract many homeopathic remedies.

IRRITATION – massage with high doses of essential oils and some base oils will aggravate the irritation, particularly skin conditions, such as psoriasis.

LOCAL INFLAMMATION – adding a strong dose of essential oil to your bath may cause you to jump out, suffering with prickly heat and redness.

SENSITISATION, allergic reaction and intense irritation.

IT IS NOT ADVISABLE to expose your skin to the sun's rays within 12 hours of dermal application of base and essential oils.

WHY SHOULD YOU AVOID
MASSAGE DURING PREGNANCY?

It is generally not considered safe to massage
pregnant women, particularly in the first trimester,
because of the high risk of complications. It is
believed that strong circular motion could stimulate
contractions. Remember, your baby is receiving your
signals and, more importantly, will absorb essential
oils via your blood stream. Some essential oils can be
harmful, and the baby could also be allergic to nuts
or other content of the base oil. It is therefore not
advisable to have a full-body massage, or even a
strong application to the feet, without your doctor's
consent, unless it is applied by a professional therapist.
However, a gentle head massage, without oils, is
acceptable, and a light, gentle, loving stroke applied to
the face and brow will relieve anxiety and release
stress. Pregnant women are also prone to back-ache,
and stroking the back, again without oils, will help
this problem.

*Gentle massage can be applied
during the later stages of pregnancy.
It can also be used as part of
a programme of natural pain
relief during labour.*

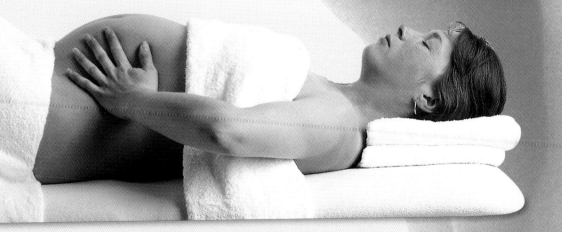

Choosing a Massage **Style**

Take your time choosing a massage style. You need to be comfortable with the therapist and the level of physical contact if you are to gain the maximum benefits from the treatment.

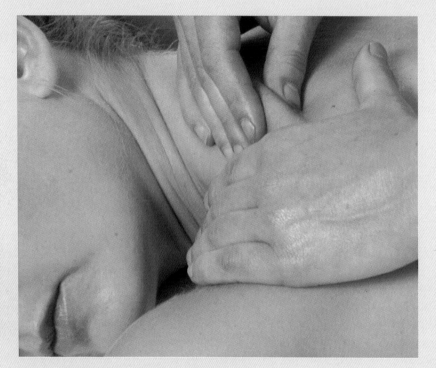

Whatever your reasons for choosing massage, it is important to feel totally comfortable with your therapist.

It is important when seeking a professional massage to know what you wish to gain from your treatment. You may have seen an advertisement or received a personal recommendation for various therapy types. These may include a massage therapist, sports injury therapist, shiatsu practitioner, Swedish masseur or aromatherapist, among many other names and titles. How do you choose the right professional therapist tailored for your present needs?

A Swedish masseur applying the style of hand movements made popular in the 18th century by the Scandinavian Per (Peter) Henrik Ling would be treating the circulatory system and improving posture, both considered crucial to body health.

Sports therapists specialise in techniques most suited for sports injury, based on increasing blood flow to the damaged site. These are often applied with more vigour and greater tissue manipulation than general massage, requiring further in-depth training and examination in physiology and anatomy.

Physical therapists may even manipulate, affecting tissues and muscles connected to the skeletal system.

Physiotherapists use either hands-on massage or, more commonly, infra-red or mechanical vibrating equipment to produce massage applications, for example:
• effleurage using mechanical vacuum suction
• kneading using a gyrator
• petrissage using ultrasound
• percussion techniques using a vibrator.

These are all proven methods to increase your blood circulation and enhance the healing process to painful joints and injuries.

Don't be embarrassed about your lack of knowledge when approaching a therapist. Ask the questions you need answering. Discuss your ailments and take your time before committing.

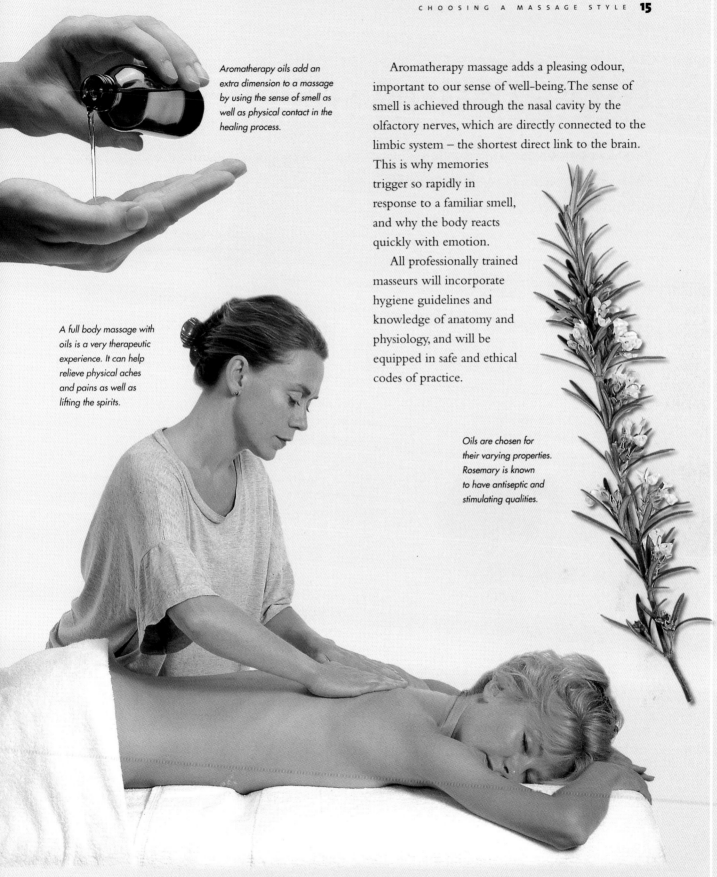

Aromatherapy oils add an extra dimension to a massage by using the sense of smell as well as physical contact in the healing process.

A full body massage with oils is a very therapeutic experience. It can help relieve physical aches and pains as well as lifting the spirits.

Aromatherapy massage adds a pleasing odour, important to our sense of well-being. The sense of smell is achieved through the nasal cavity by the olfactory nerves, which are directly connected to the limbic system – the shortest direct link to the brain. This is why memories trigger so rapidly in response to a familiar smell, and why the body reacts quickly with emotion.

All professionally trained masseurs will incorporate hygiene guidelines and knowledge of anatomy and physiology, and will be equipped in safe and ethical codes of practice.

Oils are chosen for their varying properties. Rosemary is known to have antiseptic and stimulating qualities.

Integrating Styles

It can be beneficial to combine different massage styles. For relaxation, the combination of massage with aroma induces deeper relaxation than Swedish style massage, which is more invigorating, though the aromatherapist will have many of the same massage techniques, applications and qualifications.

Some oriental therapists will use their feet as well as their hands to apply massage to their patients.

Shiatsu massage, developed in the Oriental Far East, focuses on applying direct pressure to restabilise and bring harmony to your body's vital energy meridian system, while Western styles of massage are more concerned with relaxing and soothing, aiding your physical body repair. Shiatsu methods do not rely solely on application by hands!

The study of modern-day aromatherapy is the result of the integration of external and internal alchemy, researched and popularised by the French chemist, René-Maurice Gattefossé, during the early 1920s. He had burnt his arm in his laboratory, and when he plunged it into a container of lavender oil he found that it gave astounding pain relief and that his broken skin and tissues healed rapidly.

An aromatherapy massage application will feel more relaxing and gentle than massage alone. In an aromatherapy massage, essential oils are added to the base oil. These are extracted from plants and trees – plants contain hormones and vitamins, and many have antibiotic and antiseptic properties.

Shiatsu massage relies on direct pressure to restore the body's basic harmony.

STEAM DISTILLATION

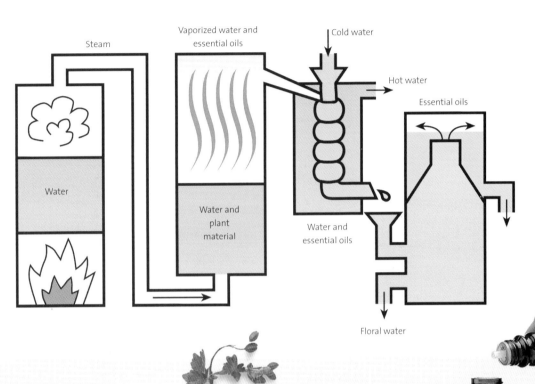

Steam · Vaporized water and essential oils · Cold water · Hot water · Essential oils · Water · Water and plant material · Water and essential oils · Floral water

Steam distillation is one of the methods used to extract essential oil. Water is heated and the steam vapour is collected in a still with the plant. The vapours produced are then cooled and collected in a vat. The source of the essential oil varies – for example, coriander is produced from the seed of the plant, while geranium is produced from both the stems and leaves of the flowering plant; ginger is produced from the root of this tropical plant; sandalwood is produced from the wood of the tree, and cedarwood from the bark of the tree; and the flowering tops of the rose bush produce rose oil. Expression is the term given to the method used for extracting citrus oils, as these are captured by squeezing the peel of the fruit.

Aromatherapy oils are concentrated and almost all of them must be mixed in a carrier oil before applying directly to the skin.

Benefits of Massage

Massage is achieved by touch. A gentle touch can capture a healing moment. Touch conveys so many messages of caring and unity – it expresses an act of kindness and compassion between one person and another, especially when given to those who do not often receive touch, such as the elderly or unwell.

A gentle squeeze to your arm as you tell a friend of your woes releases tension in your muscles and stimulates the release of chemical endorphins, the natural opiate activated within your body. This transmits a calming sensation throughout the body's nervous system, as well as stimulating your body's natural defences, reducing pain and deepening your sleep state, inducing a profound feeling of well-being and putting you in touch with your inner self. This is why you invariably sigh and relax after receiving a caring touch of empathy.

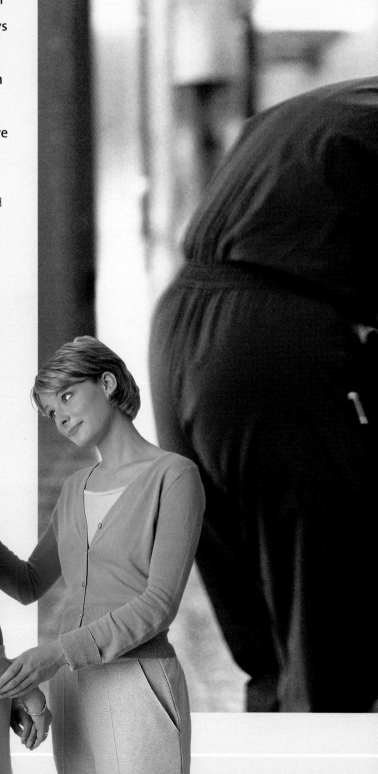

Touch can be used to calm a friend who is in distress and increase her feeling of well-being.

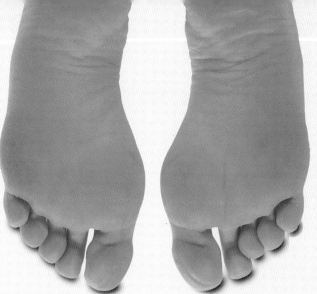

A caring touch can ease fear and offer reassurance when we are feeling insecure. Parents generally know this instinctively.

The feet are very sensitive. Reflexology is based on the zone theory that each part of the foot corresponds to another part of the body.

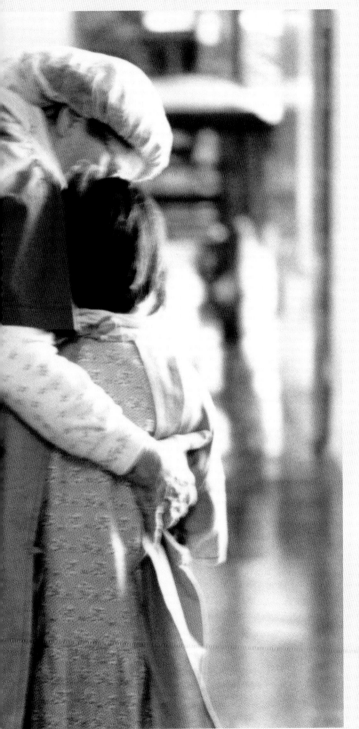

Massage tends to be applied using only the hands – fingertips, the heel of the hand, the thumbs and even the fists and forearms produce wonderful sensations in you and your recipient – but it is possible to use just about any body part to massage. The feet or knees can also be used to apply pressure and release pain from the body, while rubbing your feet gently against your partner conveys love and seduction.

We rub our shoulders when we are feeling tired, to release tension in the neck and to 'rub away' the cares of the day.

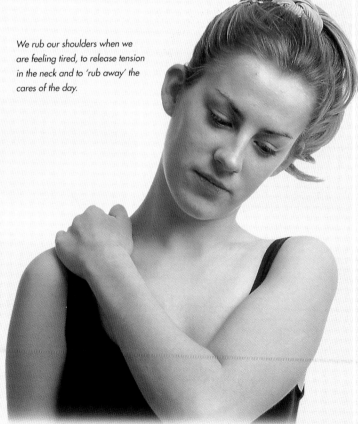

TOUCH CANNOT BE OVERRATED

Whether you receive a moment of comfort in the street or are lucky enough to experience an hour of massage on a treatment couch, the benefits are tremendous to mind, body and spirit. Massage touch enhances physical, intellectual and personal emotional growth. Massage applied by the skilled practitioner brings you in touch with the world, acknowledging that you are a part of the whole of nature's creation. Massage stimulates blood flow, increasing body temperature and the delivery of nutrients as well as eliminating waste products and heightening your senses. Massage can help the body to reduce swelling, to relax and to detoxify the muscle fibres, and to relieve other physical ailments such as tension headaches and constipation.

The word 'touch' can conjure up many pictures in your mind. It may suggest advertising posters that encourage you to reach out to your neighbour and bring unity to the human race; or an advertisement for a skin-care product with which you can seduce and pamper your own body, bringing you total relaxation. What does massage touch convey to you? Ask yourself again later today, tomorrow, and next week, and see how your response varies with your daily lifestyle. Note the effects of how you react on a day-to-day basis and, more importantly, see how the regular use of massage in your life helps you to grow and develop the spiritual side of your nature.

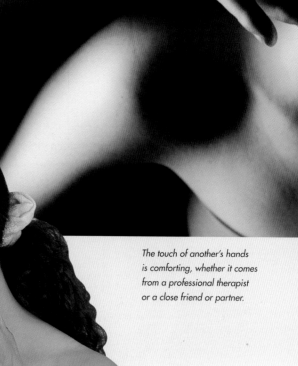

The touch of another's hands is comforting, whether it comes from a professional therapist or a close friend or partner.

Applying face creams with a gentle circular motion gives skin a mini-massage that stimulates blood flow.

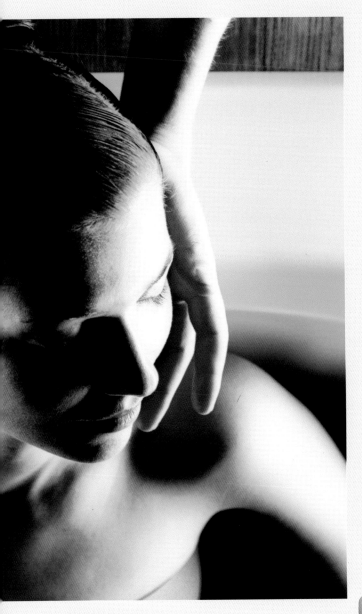

*Massage treats the whole person –
physically, mentally, emotionally
and spiritually.*

more of massage really allows you to slow down and switch off, both mentally and physically, from the pressures of society.

On a physical level, massage treats the whole person, releasing tension from the mind and the muscles, communicating through caring touch, imparting inner peace and tranquillity. When you are receiving a massage, you may find that you tend to drift away into your own personal paradise.

When you give a massage, energy is transmitted, touching your inner spiritual self. When massage is given with compassion, healing takes place at high levels. A spiritual level is reached through the rejuvenation of your chi, your vital life energy. Chi is an unseen force of nature that runs through your body in the same way as the visible arteries and veins. Massage promotes self-awareness and treats the mind, body and spirit, enabling you to achieve a truly holistic state of homeostasis, returning balance and harmony to yourself.

WHY HAVE A MASSAGE?

If you have a busy, stressful lifestyle, you will really appreciate a little time to yourself. There are many ways in which you can take time out, such as going to the theatre or cinema, an exercise class, or swimming – indeed numerous leisure activities are available to you; yet they still require you to use your body physically or concentrate mentally, or both, often adding more pressure to your already increasingly pressurised daily life. One hour or

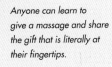

*Anyone can learn to
give a massage and share
the gift that is literally at
their fingertips.*

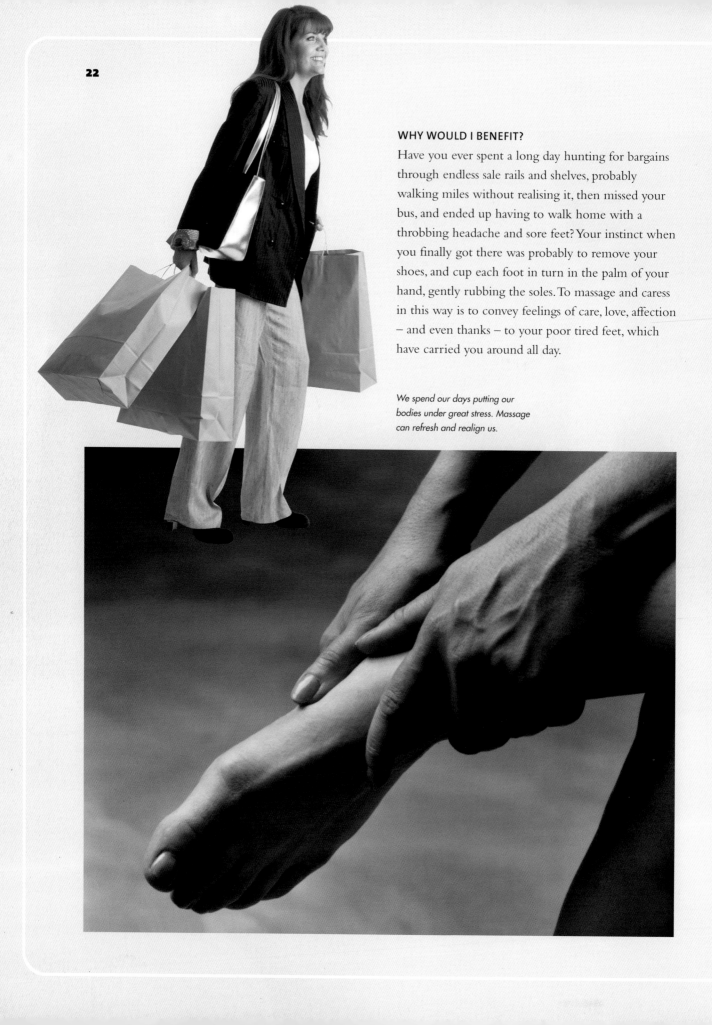

WHY WOULD I BENEFIT?

Have you ever spent a long day hunting for bargains through endless sale rails and shelves, probably walking miles without realising it, then missed your bus, and ended up having to walk home with a throbbing headache and sore feet? Your instinct when you finally got there was probably to remove your shoes, and cup each foot in turn in the palm of your hand, gently rubbing the soles. To massage and caress in this way is to convey feelings of care, love, affection – and even thanks – to your poor tired feet, which have carried you around all day.

We spend our days putting our bodies under great stress. Massage can refresh and realign us.

THE BENEFITS OF MASSAGE

Everyone has their own reasons for trying massage, and not everyone will react in the same way to it.
However, everyone can benefit in some way, be it physically, mentally, emotionally or spiritually.
For example, you might decide you need a monthly aromatherapy session to ease your stress coupled
with other occasional therapies to treat specific physical problems.

It is deeply relaxing

It helps you to slow down and destress

It is soothing and caring

It helps to reduce anxiety and stress

It treats the whole person – mind, body and spirit

It imparts a sense of well-being

It makes you aware of your body, including any ailments

It aids pain relief

It increases the blood flow, improving poor circulation and sending blood to a damaged site to aid repair

It releases the body's endorphins – the natural opiates that induce drowsiness, sleep, and deep relaxation

It aids digestion and the efficient disposal of waste products

It helps eliminate waste from the lymphatic system and detoxify the body

It releases muscle tension and aids the release of toxins from the muscle fibres, freeing blockages

It encourages chi to flow freely through the meridian system

It brings fresh blood to any congested areas, freeing waste and feeding nutrients and oxygen

It helps to remove dead cells from the skin by exfoliation, improving blood supply to deeper levels of the skin and to the connective tissues

It improves sleep quality

It strengthens the body's immune system

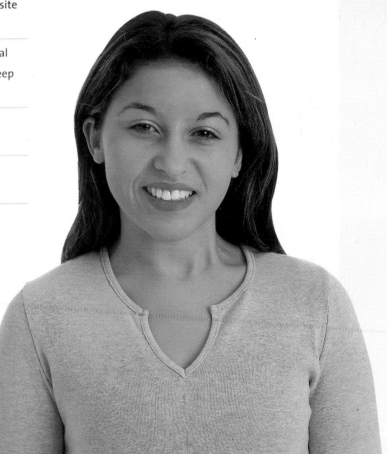

*Regular massage can help you stay
physically and mentally ready for
anything. It not only heals, but is also
a way of protecting against stress.*

Massage with Affection

Show someone that you care. Tell someone you love them, not with words but with unspoken communication. Show them with touch – show them with massage.

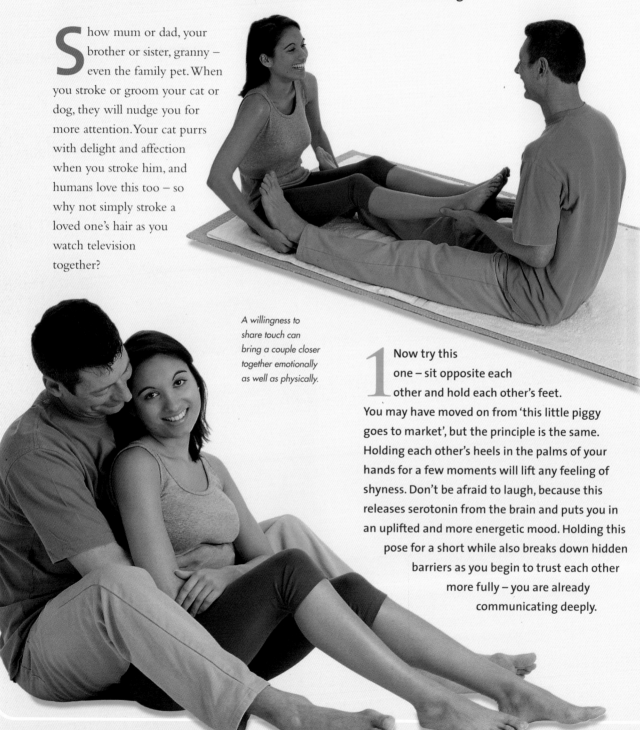

Show mum or dad, your brother or sister, granny – even the family pet. When you stroke or groom your cat or dog, they will nudge you for more attention. Your cat purrs with delight and affection when you stroke him, and humans love this too – so why not simply stroke a loved one's hair as you watch television together?

A willingness to share touch can bring a couple closer together emotionally as well as physically.

1 Now try this one – sit opposite each other and hold each other's feet. You may have moved on from 'this little piggy goes to market', but the principle is the same. Holding each other's heels in the palms of your hands for a few moments will lift any feeling of shyness. Don't be afraid to laugh, because this releases serotonin from the brain and puts you in an uplifted and more energetic mood. Holding this pose for a short while also breaks down hidden barriers as you begin to trust each other more fully – you are already communicating deeply.

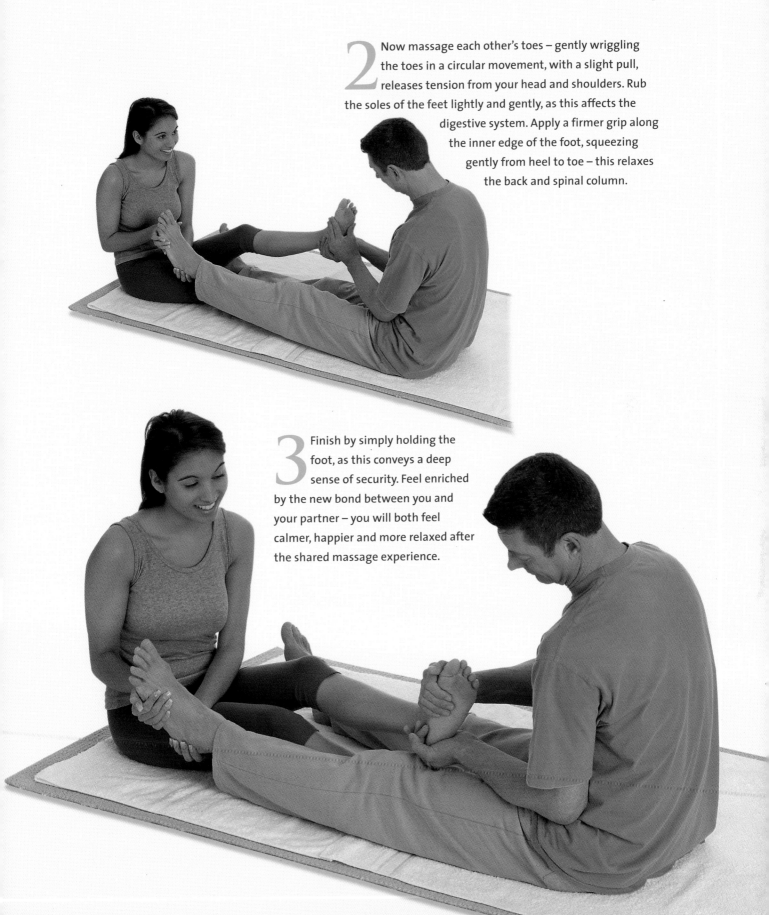

2 Now massage each other's toes – gently wriggling the toes in a circular movement, with a slight pull, releases tension from your head and shoulders. Rub the soles of the feet lightly and gently, as this affects the digestive system. Apply a firmer grip along the inner edge of the foot, squeezing gently from heel to toe – this relaxes the back and spinal column.

3 Finish by simply holding the foot, as this conveys a deep sense of security. Feel enriched by the new bond between you and your partner – you will both feel calmer, happier and more relaxed after the shared massage experience.

The effects of **Massage** on the **Body**

The human body is a physical, feeling organism that responds to external physical influences, such as massage, with a range of reactions.

You tried massaging gently, but your partner's skin has gone all red! Don't panic, because this is good. What has happened is called erythema – flushing of the skin caused by dilation of the blood capillaries in the dermis. In other words, you have stimulated the blood flow to the surface veins, increasing the oxygen levels in your blood. This in turn increases the nutrients that nourish the body, and also encourages the lymphatic waste system to work more rhythmically, releasing the toxins from the body more efficiently.

Don't be frightened to apply firm pressure when giving a massage. You need to work not just on the surface but also on the tissues beneath.

WHY DO YOU SOMETIMES FEEL COLD AFTER A MASSAGE?

Massage treats both the body and the spirit. One physical reason why you feel cold is that cardiac output decreases during massage. One spiritual reason is that negative energy is released from your body, sometimes causing you to experience a shivery physical reaction.

How does massage benefit the body in daily life? How does massage react with the body? What changes take place?

Look at how both your mind and body react when you are faced with making a conscious decision. Perhaps someone is challenging you in an offensive manner. How shall you best react? Should you choose to stay and fight, or should you turn and run? And why, when the situation is over, do you feel an incredible rush to the solar plexus region of your gut, and experience a surge of nausea?

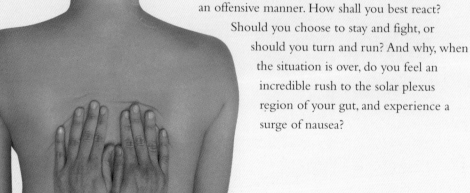

Releasing negative energy or emotions can cause a chill feeling, so dress warmly after a massage session.

What happens in this situation is that the brain stimulates hormonal changes in the body's endocrine system, producing the hormones most commonly associated with stress – adrenalin and noradrenalin, secreted by the adrenal gland. These small-sized neurotransmitter messengers have a huge impact. The muscles tense and the heart-rate increases to carry extra blood to the muscles as they prepare themselves for action, raising the blood pressure. The extra blood supply requires more oxygen so the breathing becomes more rapid. The mouth becomes dry as the digestive system switches off temporarily, relaxing the smooth muscle in the intestinal wall. The liver releases glucose to provide energy. The immune system slows down, and you often sweat in anticipation of the external reaction.

Following all that, is it any wonder that massage would convey a caring, sympathetic, physical touch to your body? In relaxing your parasympathetic nervous system, you send signals throughout your body, enabling your heart-rate and breathing to self-regulate, aiding your digestion once more, and returning the body balance and harmony, which is known as homeostasis.

The benefits of massage are so all-embracing because it is a holistic therapy, treating the body as a complex of interrelated systems, not looking merely at the symptoms of individual ailments.

To understand massage, it is useful to have a basic knowledge and understanding of the body systems and how they work together.

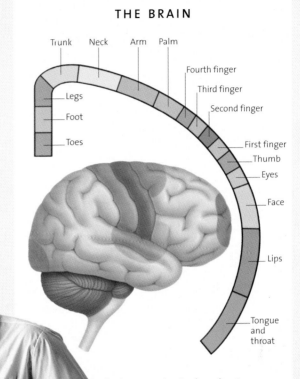

THE BRAIN

Trunk Neck Arm Palm

Legs

Foot

Toes

Fourth finger
Third finger
Second finger
First finger
Thumb
Eyes
Face
Lips
Tongue and throat

The brain and spinal cord get messages from the various sensitive areas of the body (the degree of sensitivity of each is shown by the amount of coloured area in the key) and then transmit instructions around the body in response. You can see that the fingers, palms and face are very sensitive areas of the body, the lips, tongue and throat even more so.

Changes in hormone and oxygen levels occur during a massage. Make sure you are grounded before you venture back out into the world.

How the **Body** Works

The systems of the body are interconnected — a problem in one area might have causes elsewhere. Only by understanding the complex relationships between the muscles, skeleton, cardiovascular system, nervous system, lymphatic system and digestion can we begin to cure our ills.

BODY WORKS

Movement is brought about by muscle contraction controlled by signals from the brain, which are then processed by the central nervous system.

Muscles work by contraction. Each individual fibre contracts fully, and the fibres slide over each other to make the muscle length shorter. The muscles have different shapes according to the role they play in the process of movement.

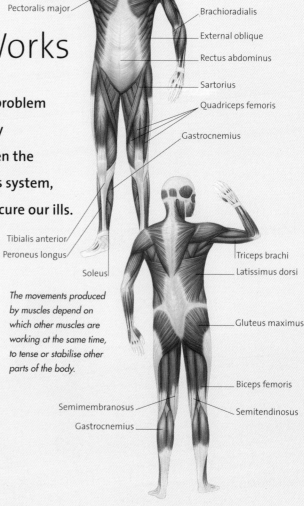

Biceps brachi

Pectoralis major

Sterno- Cleidomastoid

Deltoid

Brachioradialis

External oblique

Rectus abdominus

Sartorius

Quadriceps femoris

Gastrocnemius

Tibialis anterior

Peroneus longus

Soleus

The movements produced by muscles depend on which other muscles are working at the same time, to tense or stabilise other parts of the body.

Triceps brachi

Latissimus dorsi

Gluteus maximus

Biceps femoris

Semimembranosus

Semitendinosus

Gastrocnemius

MUSCLE STRUCTURE

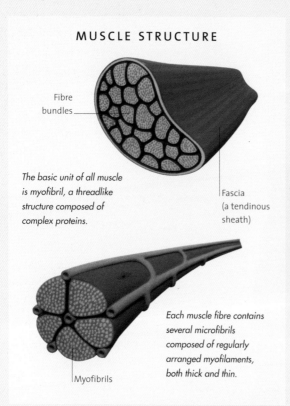

Fibre bundles

The basic unit of all muscle is myofibril, a threadlike structure composed of complex proteins.

Fascia (a tendinous sheath)

Each muscle fibre contains several microfibrils composed of regularly arranged myofilaments, both thick and thin.

Myofibrils

The muscles work in pairs — as one lengthens, the other contracts, allowing movement. Elasticity enables the muscles to return to their normal state between conscious movement. Muscles take their energy from the body's supply of oxygen, glycogen and fat, and produce waste products of carbon dioxide, lactic acid, heat and water.

The body is held in a permanent state of readiness, resulting in muscle fatigue and muscle tension. The pain that you feel in your muscles is the result of a build-up of sticky lactic acid between the fibres, which prevents them crossing over each other smoothly. You need help to expel the waste product from your muscles, and this is provided by some of the other internal body systems.

WASTE AND TOXINS

Elimination of waste products is dealt with not only by the digestive and urinary functions, but also by the lymphatic system. The lymphatic system does not operate from the pulsing heartbeat, but acts independently, relying on muscle contraction along with gravity and passive movement to protect the body from the invasion of foreign bacteria.

Imagine a train running along miles of railway track, which has stations at intervals – some major stations, and some minor ones. When the lymphatic system is working efficiently, waste products are moved from one tiny vessel to the next, as if passing through the carriages on the train. When the lymph reaches a lymph node, it is like the train reaching a station; and like a train off-loading its passengers, the lymph off-loads bacteria, dead cells and other harmful substances. If the lymphatic system is not working efficiently, however, the lymph nodes are like stations trying to operate with a reduced staff – tension is created by backlogs, the systems fail to work properly and normal service is suspended. When this happens in the lymphatic nodes, you will feel unwell and you may find that your glands are swollen.

When you feel unwell and have a temperature, it is unwise to massage affected areas as you could increase the blockages rather than free them. Trained therapists know when massage is inadvisable.

The lymphatic system also transports dietary fats from the small intestine into the blood supply and interstitial fluid, draining the tissues of proteins and returning them to the circulation via the cardio-vascular system.

As it runs alongside the blood flow, the speed of flow relies on the heart rate, again showing how the body organs and accessory organs are dependent upon one another.

The lymphatic system uses muscle contraction to play its part in the elimination of waste from the body.

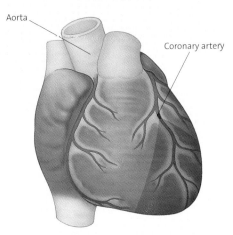

THE HEART

Aorta

Coronary artery

The dual pumping system of the heart is dependent on the cardiac muscles of which it is made for receiving oxygenated blood and transporting it around the body.

RESTLESS HEART

Energy levels rely largely on intake of food. Energy is not only needed to exert external muscle projection. Internally, the cardio-vascular system operates like the transport industry. Its function includes a 'distribution service' to deliver oxygen and nutrients and remove unwanted carbon dioxide and waste products from the cells, balancing product levels in the body and maintaining pH acid balance in the cells and tissues. The lymphatic system assists in the removal of bacteria and waste products.

The heart acts as the distribution manager. It weighs about 250–350g (9–12oz) in adults, is around the size of a clenched fist, and is a four-chambered pump. Its function is to receive oxygenated blood, which is then transported to the muscles, tissues and organs. It is supported by the respiratory system – deoxygenated blood is pumped into the lungs, where carbon dioxide and oxygen are exchanged. The heart is self-stimulating, and continues its never-ending job even when you are sleeping.

SKIN AND BONES

The skeletal system – together with the muscles, tendons and ligaments – is what enables the human body to defy gravity and stand upright.

The function of the skeletal system is to protect the internal organs, assist movement, and support and hold rigid the anatomical structure. It is even involved in the production of marrow and calcium.

Covering the body mass is the largest of the accessory organs – the skin. The skin is a huge expanse of protective, waterproof covering – but there is more to it than this. The skin, aided by the nervous system, allows you to experience pleasure and pain and to detect the gentlest breeze, hot or cold. The skin has an appearance that reflects your inner state of health – bright and glowing when you are well, dull and drawn when you are not. The receptor nerve endings found beneath the skin communicate a great deal – these are what tell you the difference between a loving kiss and a punch on the nose! Touch is the primary sense, which we so often take for granted. Massage is your gift of touch.

The skin protects deeper levels of your anatomy, and also shields you from harmful penetration by ultra-violet light and bacteria and from physical abrasion. If the skin were not waterproof, you would swell like a piece of bread soaked in water when you took a bath; yet when base oil and essential oil are massaged into the skin, they are absorbed through the hair follicles, allowing the essential oil to target the organ with which it has an affinity.

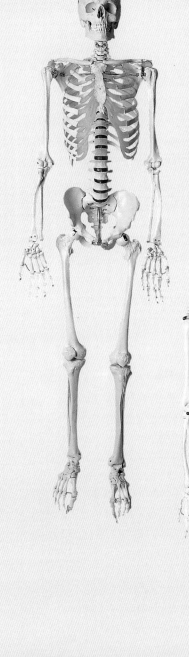

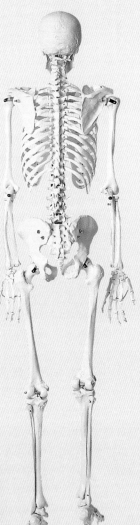

A healthy structure of tendons and muscles is important to our posture because of its influence on the position of our bones.

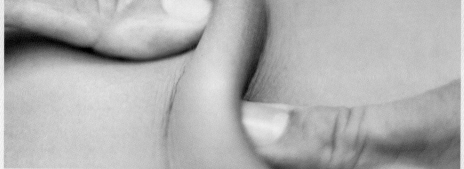

Massage can help to relieve tension in muscles which allows the skeletal system to realign, thus relieving pain and discomfort.

The skin also assists in the regulation of body temperature. When you are hot, moisture is brought to the surface of the skin in the form of sweat to cool you down. The sudorific (sweat) glands and the sebaceous oil glands also help in the elimination of excess toxins from the body. When you are cold, you feel the sensation of 'goose bumps' – these are your hairs standing up to provide protection from the cold by trapping in your body heat.

Your skin has three main layers, which in turn subdivide further.

Just below the dermis there is adipose tissue – the fat cells. As these cells collect and bump into one another, they compact and attach to the subcutaneous level of tissue that begins the process of creating your skin.

The loose connective tissue, with collagen and elastic fibres, interlaces. The reticular dense coarse connective fibres intermix to form the structure. The structure of the skin is thicker on the lateral and dorsal body, but thinner on the eyelids, enabling the skin to crease rapidly with eye movement. The papillary capillaries, with their good strong blood supply, leave two dermis layers projecting into the outer level of the skin, known as the epidermis.

The epidermis consists of five layers which develop in stages, each taking two to four weeks to reach the surface. In skin conditions such as psoriasis, however, this can take as little as four days – the skin is produced too quickly, and then has a shorter life span and less activity.

The basale, or germinative, layer is the deepest of these five layers, known more commonly as the true skin. New cells form, and together with the cells still intact they create discs known as 'merkles discs', some

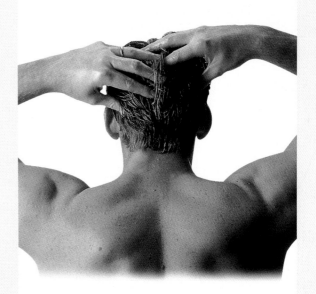

SKIN STRUCTURE

There is more to the skin than the outer layer we can see. Its complex structure is part of the body's overall regulatory system.

Creams and oils applied to the outer layer of skin are absorbed into the tissues beneath the surface.

eight to ten layers deep. These are sensitive to touch, and are known as the 'prickle' layer.

In the next three to five cell layers, which are gradually pushed out towards the surface, the cells become impregnated with keratin, which makes the skin waterproof and is the major constituent of hair and nails.

Then comes the 'lucid' layer, the clearish layer that is thicker on the soles of the feet and the palms of the hands.

The horny layer, which is the top or outer surface layer, is made up of some 25 to 30 rows of flat dead cells which are packed full of keratin, providing you with a waterproof barrier against the elements of light and heat, bacteria and chemicals.

Massage for General **Well-being, Injury** and **Illness**

While the benefits of massage for physical ailments, such as sports injury or strained muscles, are well-known, massage can also be used to treat a whole range of other problems that at first it might be difficult to imagine could be improved by physical manipulation.

The human body is a complex structure, so it is not perhaps so surprising that in addition to the obvious medical problems massage can help, it can also play a role in alleviating such conditions as depression, nasal congestion, digestive disorders as well as muscle and joint problems.

A competent massage therapist will always take comprehensive notes about a patient's past medical history as well as details about their lifestyle to provide pointers to any underlying problems that might not be immediately apparent. A note will also be made of any conventional treatment or medication being taken. A thorough but gentle investigation will usually reveal which areas need particular attention before the massage begins. A professional therapist will also turn away patients for whom their particular form of massage would not be appropriate.

The following case histories show how massage in its various forms can be used to treat a variety of ailments and that even where it cannot offer a cure, it can relieve symptoms and so boost self-esteem and improve quality of life. The case histories cover a range of ages, both male and female.

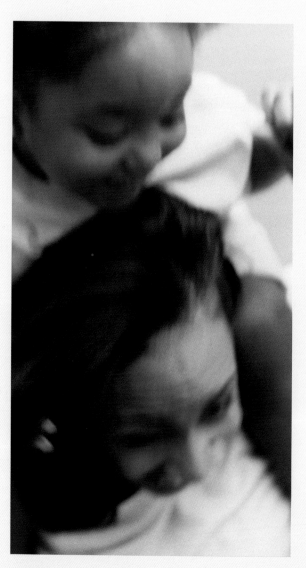

Massage can be used to alleviate symptoms caused by the stresses and strains of daily living, without resorting to drugs.

CASE HISTORY 1

AGE 29

SEX Female

OCCUPATION Secretary

REASON FOR CONSULTATION/SYMPTOMS
Chronic asthma, heartburn and constipation, very overweight, migraines, mood swings, wants to become pregnant

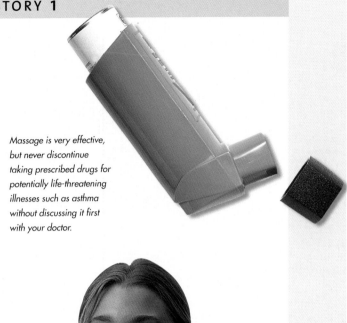

Massage is very effective, but never discontinue taking prescribed drugs for potentially life-threatening illnesses such as asthma without discussing it first with your doctor.

First treatment During first treatment it was found that she had blocked sinus, irritable bowel syndrome, left knee-joint wear and tear, muscle tension and crystals of lactic acid build-up in shoulder areas. It was clearly audible that there was chronic asthma.

Following treatment she described herself as feeling quite odd and very relaxed, without pain to chest or knee.

Subsequent treatment Returned twice-weekly for two months and then for a regular monthly massage for well-being following recovery of all ailments. Treatment continued throughout most of her recent pregnancy and she has now returned with baby for 'mum and baby' massage. Still a little overweight, no longer on daily asthma medication – only taken as or when required.

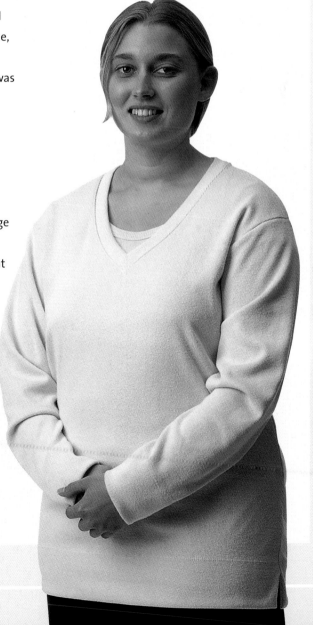

Massage treats the whole person, so it can be used to relieve symptoms caused by a variety of problems all in the same treatment session.

CASE HISTORY 2

AGE 45

SEX Male

OCCUPATION Solicitor

REASON FOR CONSULTATION/SYMPTOMS
Severe psoriasis for 20 years, fed up with this
and very stressed with work commitments.

Treatments Following lengthy discussion with
regard to symptoms, diet and lifestyle, skin was
patch-tested for oil application. Most of the body
at this stage unsuitable for dermal application as
psoriasis affects skin by rapid cell growth. Loose
clothing was worn for first six treatments at
seven-ten day intervals; built up to two-weekly to
three-weekly intervals and eventually to present
five-six week intervals. Applications now dermal.
Treatments invariably use anger-
management skills with breath control
and talk therapy, though he is now far
happier with his family life and more
tolerant of the nature of his work. He
is much calmer, which has shown great
impact on his daily life and is reflected
in the slowing down of his skin cell
reproduction. He has received
treatment for 20 months.

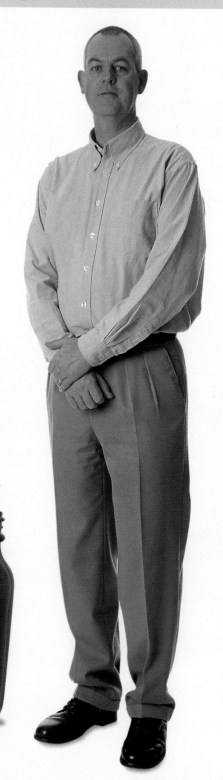

*Essential oils are very strong and must be
applied with care, particularly where
there are visible problems with the skin*

CASE HISTORY 3

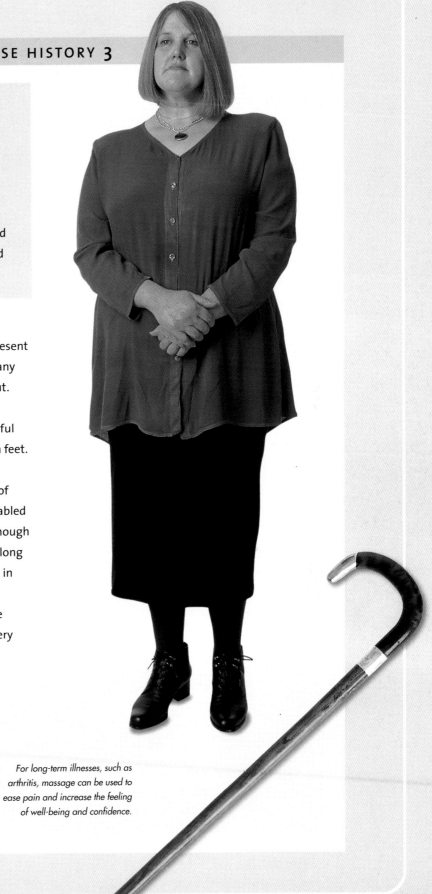

AGE 50

SEX Female

OCCUPATION University Secretary

REASON FOR CONSULTATION/SYMPTOMS
Disabled. Severe arthritis. Difficulty in walking, general body pain. Partially sighted and partially deaf. Irritable. Overweight and signs of depression.

First treatment Lot of erythema (flushing) present in the back along with great pain. Visually many broken veins. Muscle tension solid throughout. Left leg very painful with heat present. Very limited neck or joint movement. Left hip painful and mostly immobile. Unbearable pain felt in feet.

Subsequent treatment Following 11 months of treatment she has just been declined her disabled driver badge! She can now walk unaided, although shuffling still on waking and after sitting for long periods. Still suffering with intermittent pain in soles of feet and occasionally pain in back. Generally very much improved. Now in stable relationship too! Life is looking and feeling very much better for her in general.

For long-term illnesses, such as arthritis, massage can be used to ease pain and increase the feeling of well-being and confidence.

CASE HISTORY 4

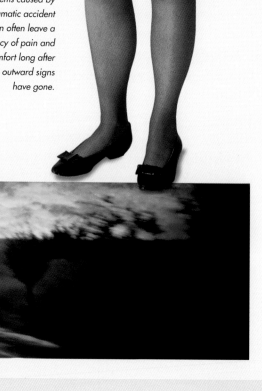

AGE 45

SEX Female

OCCUPATION School Bursar

REASON FOR CONSULTATION/SYMPTOMS
Trauma following horrific road traffic
accident, severe whiplash, blackouts, amnesia,
vomiting and diarrhoea, pain to entire body
and hallucinations.

First treatment Passive effleurage revealed
bruising and possible disc damage. Tissue damage
to neck and shoulder region. Manual lymphatic
drainage massage to scalp area applied. Leg
mobility affected. She fell into a deep relaxed sleep
for the first time since RTA some weeks earlier.

Subsequent treatment Repeating massage
treatments to posterior only every four days for
one month and then weekly for a further two
weeks, then introducing front and back body
massage weekly for a further four weeks. In most
part full recovery, however still suffering from
occasional whiplash and psychological trauma
though to far less extent.

*Problems caused by
a traumatic accident
can often leave a
legacy of pain and
discomfort long after
the outward signs
have gone.*

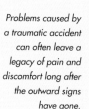

CASE HISTORY 5

AGE 42

SEX Male

OCCUPATION Accountant – self-employed

REASON FOR CONSULTATION/SYMPTOMS
Sports injury

Prompt attention to a sports injury can relieve the swelling that causes pain and can lead to a speedy recovery without the need for drugs.

First treatment Came with a sports injury five years ago for very inflamed knee cap.

Subsequent treatment Varied over years to treat further sports injuries as keen squash player, footballer and ju-jitsu instructor. Massage given for injuries when requested, and massage for well-being on a monthly basis.

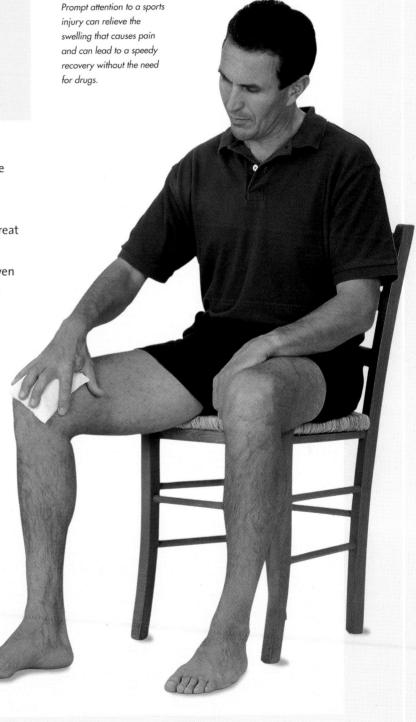

CASE HISTORY 6

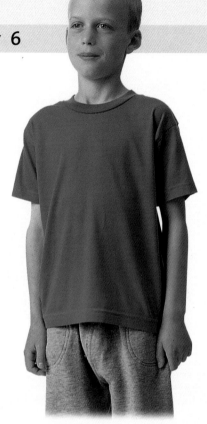

AGE 10

SEX Male

OCCUPATION Junior School pupil

REASON FOR CONSULTATION/SYMPTOMS
Pains to joints

First treatment Massage to lower limbs. No inflammation present though mobility painful. Advised agreement with general practitioner that problem was growing pains.

Subsequent treatment Follow-up appointment not kept as pain relief after first visit sustained. Has returned twice more for similar pains in leg and in hip. Massage applied to localised sites, pain relief immediate on following visits too.

Massage to areas of localised pain is particularly useful with children for whom medication may be unwanted or ill-advised.

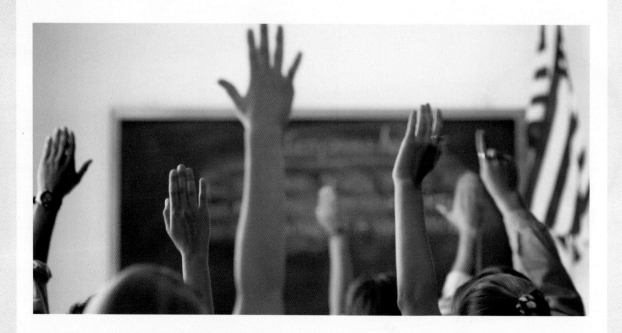

CASE HISTORY 7

AGE 70

SEX Female

OCCUPATION Housewife

REASON FOR CONSULTATION/SYMPTOMS
Parkinsons diagnosed seven years earlier.
Migraine. Weak ankles. Coordination
difficulty. Poor sleep pattern. Arthritis to right
hip. Dyspepsia. Sinus irritation. Panic and
anxiety attacks. Recently widowed.

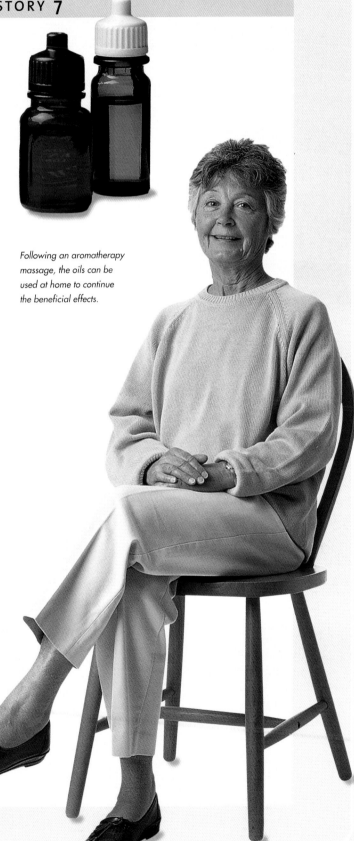

*Following an aromatherapy
massage, the oils can be
used at home to continue
the beneficial effects.*

First treatment Full body massage applied,
concentrating on head, legs and feet. Some pain
relief felt generally, though a long way to go for
stability of pain relief.

Subsequent treatment Four weekly massages,
followed by four fortnightly and then continuous
monthly. Continual progress was made with her
taking a trip away for the week less than six
months from commencement. Confidence and
walking greatly improved. Attacks caused progress
to suffer from time to time but always picked up
again following treatment, with the added
essential oils helping to stimulate mind and body
progress. After 11 months, massage applied at 6-8
week intervals, plus Christmas and birthday treats
as presents from her family members.

Creating the right Atmosphere

Make yourself comfortable before your massage begins.

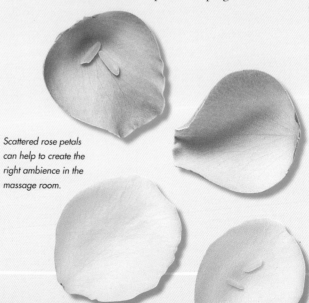

How do you create the right atmosphere for a massage session? Lighting, temperature, furnishings and aroma all play their part.

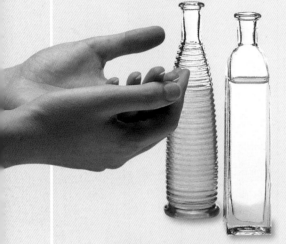

Choose oils that have positive associations or the potential good will be lost.

C reating the right atmosphere for massage is not only fun, it will also extend your enjoyment of both giving and receiving message. It need not take long to achieve – with a bit of imagination your living room can be transformed into an Indian temple. Throw drapes, scarves and cushions around your room or floor space. Choose natural fabrics where possible.

Colour is proven to play an important part in your mood and confidence levels, and the absorption of the colour spectrum stimulates your chakras – the body's invisible energy centres.

Buy yourself some flowers with a strong scent, such as roses, lilies or narcissi. Be extravagant and scatter rose petals across your room or bed.

Dim the lights or light candles. Warm the room, which must well-ventilated if you are using essential oils, but do not massage in a direct draught.

Consider the stage set. Are you suitably dressed to project the image you wish to for the occasion?

Make sure you have all the props and equipment you will need. A firm massagé couch is preferable, but is not often available in the home. You may choose to lie on the end of a firm bed, although the height may be uncomfortable for the giver of massage. The floor, being firm, is good, too, or you could consider using your dining room table, covered with a blanket to protect it.

You will want to lie on a soft blanket, towel or sheet, and have two large towels to cover yourself. Soft music is an aid to relaxation as this helps you to calm your mind. You will need base oil or talcum powder to avoid friction burning. Dimming the lights, using a table lamp or lighting candles creates a more relaxed, subdued atmosphere. Unplug the

Scattered rose petals can help to create the right ambience in the massage room.

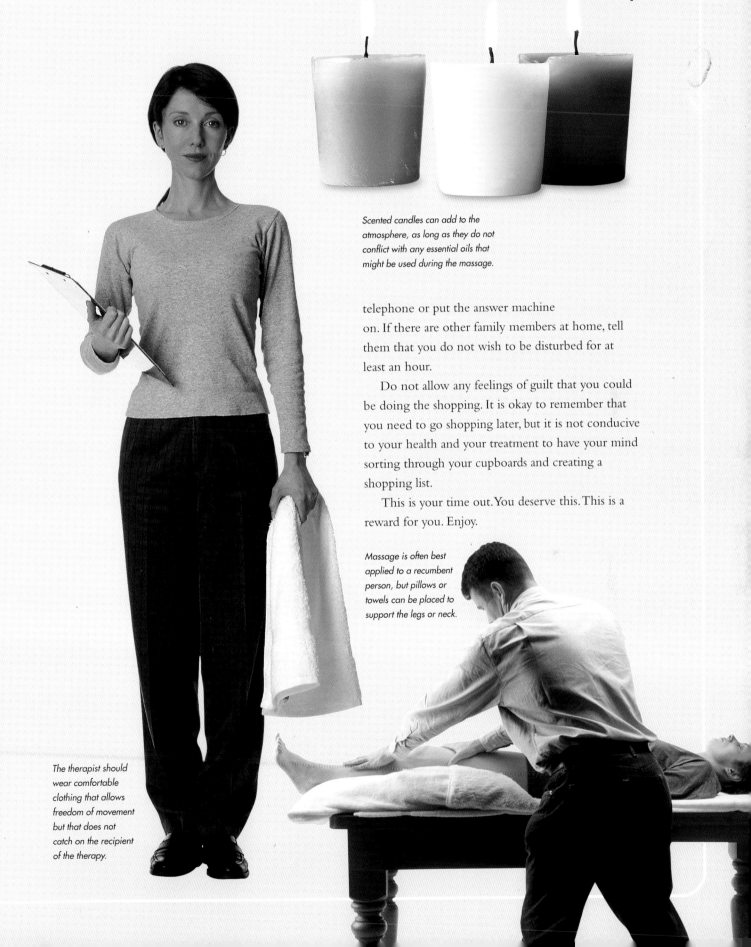

Scented candles can add to the atmosphere, as long as they do not conflict with any essential oils that might be used during the massage.

telephone or put the answer machine on. If there are other family members at home, tell them that you do not wish to be disturbed for at least an hour.

Do not allow any feelings of guilt that you could be doing the shopping. It is okay to remember that you need to go shopping later, but it is not conducive to your health and your treatment to have your mind sorting through your cupboards and creating a shopping list.

This is your time out. You deserve this. This is a reward for you. Enjoy.

Massage is often best applied to a recumbent person, but pillows or towels can be placed to support the legs or neck.

The therapist should wear comfortable clothing that allows freedom of movement but that does not catch on the recipient of the therapy.

Basic **Techniques**

A massage includes a combination of techniques designed to work the muscles and tissues in various ways, depending on where they are and what benefit is desired.

When applying massage techniques, ensure that your body weight is behind your stroke. This will not only produce a deeper, more rhythmic flow to your 'partner' (that is, the recipient of the massage), it will prevent you as the giver from feeling tired out, and instead you will feel energised. If you watch any top professional at work, they always appear to glide effortlessly and tirelessly in mesmerising motion. World-class swimmers smoothly push aside the water with each stroke; they do not punch at the water, as this would waste valuable time and energy.

Massage strokes must be applied firmly and rhythmically. If they are too hard and they will be painful; too light and they will tickle and irritate.

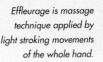

Effleurage is massage technique applied by light stroking movements of the whole hand.

Effleurage

Effleurage, meaning to 'skim over', is a light stroking movement of the whole hand, and can be used all over the body. Body weight can be introduced to exert pressure, though this should be kept minimal at the beginning until you connect with your partner, and graduate back to a light pressure at the conclusion of the massage, as you remove your connection. It will also give you information, as you gain experience, about your partner's health.

Effleurage helps venous blood flow and lymphatic drainage. The depth of the stroke influences the manipulation of the fluids to the superficial vessels. Effleurage is found to promote the most beneficial psychological and physical relaxation, and prepares the muscles for deeper manipulation.

To apply effleurage, your hands should be relaxed, with the fingers touching and the thumbs slightly apart. Begin by stroking gently, moving your hand rhythmically away from you and back toward you. As you develop the feel of the stroke, alternate each hand, so one hand is moving forward and the other drawing back, keeping contact with the body. These strokes can be performed all over the body. Smooth the skin lightly in the direction of the heart.

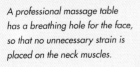

A professional massage table has a breathing hole for the face, so that no unnecessary strain is placed on the neck muscles.

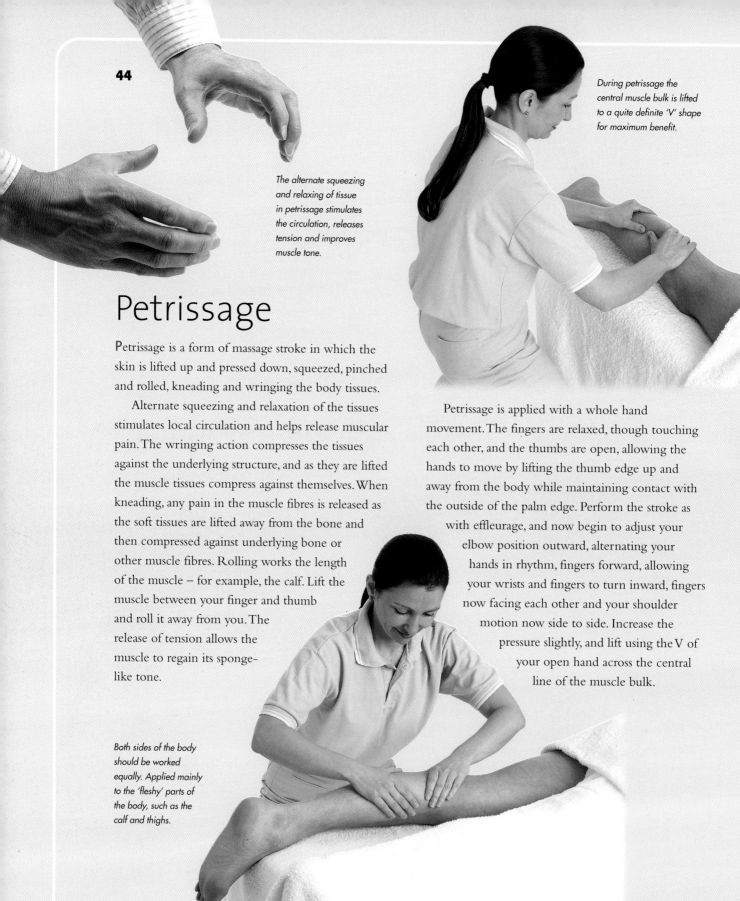

The alternate squeezing and relaxing of tissue in petrissage stimulates the circulation, releases tension and improves muscle tone.

During petrissage the central muscle bulk is lifted to a quite definite 'V' shape for maximum benefit.

Petrissage

Petrissage is a form of massage stroke in which the skin is lifted up and pressed down, squeezed, pinched and rolled, kneading and wringing the body tissues.

Alternate squeezing and relaxation of the tissues stimulates local circulation and helps release muscular pain. The wringing action compresses the tissues against the underlying structure, and as they are lifted the muscle tissues compress against themselves. When kneading, any pain in the muscle fibres is released as the soft tissues are lifted away from the bone and then compressed against underlying bone or other muscle fibres. Rolling works the length of the muscle – for example, the calf. Lift the muscle between your finger and thumb and roll it away from you. The release of tension allows the muscle to regain its sponge-like tone.

Petrissage is applied with a whole hand movement. The fingers are relaxed, though touching each other, and the thumbs are open, allowing the hands to move by lifting the thumb edge up and away from the body while maintaining contact with the outside of the palm edge. Perform the stroke as with effleurage, and now begin to adjust your elbow position outward, alternating your hands in rhythm, fingers forward, allowing your wrists and fingers to turn inward, fingers now facing each other and your shoulder motion now side to side. Increase the pressure slightly, and lift using the V of your open hand across the central line of the muscle bulk.

Both sides of the body should be worked equally. Applied mainly to the 'fleshy' parts of the body, such as the calf and thighs.

Kneading

Kneading is applied with a whole hand movement, with fingers relaxed but touching, and thumbs open. Lightly grasp the muscle and skin, picking up and squeezing the contours of the body beneath, still using your whole hand. Release with one hand as you apply the other. Develop a rhythmic swaying from side to side with your body weight as you apply your alternating hands.

CAUTION

Avoid squeezing with the fingertips as this may hurt your partner.

Kneading is perhaps what most people think of when they hear the word 'massage', but it is just one of a range of techniques for applying pressure.

Wringing

Wringing is used on larger areas of the body such as the torso, thighs and calves. Use the whole hand – palm and fingers – and with a lifting motion draw the skin toward you with one hand and away from you with the other. Lift the skin as you do so to avoid friction and to manipulate stimulation to internal organs. Release the pressure and reverse the action, keeping contact with a push-lift, slide-pull action. For small muscles, it is possible to wring with just a thumb movement.

CAUTION

Release of tension takes place on both physical and emotional levels. Your partner may experience overwhelming feelings of emotion, ranging from tears of release to sighs of relief.

Wringing involves the whole hand – both palm and fingers. Draw the skin towards you with one hand and away from you with the other.

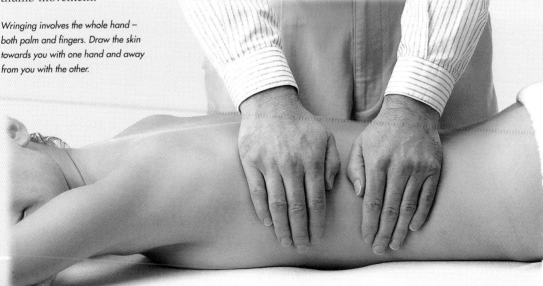

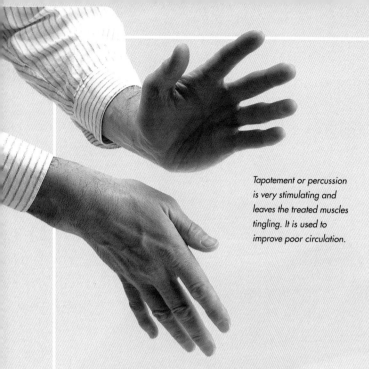

Tapotement or percussion is very stimulating and leaves the treated muscles tingling. It is used to improve poor circulation.

Cupping

This technique involves making a cup shape with your hands and using a controlled, flicking movement on the rounder contours of the body.

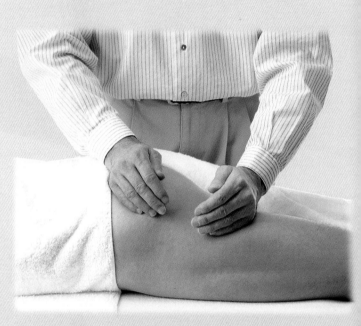

Tapotement

Tapotement is sometimes called percussion because of the wonderful sounds it produces. It includes cupping, hacking, vibration and tapping.

The body part being treated is struck with soft blows of the hand propelled by wrist action, stimulating and promoting muscle reflexes. It can be applied to areas of poor circulation, lymphatic drainage or muscle tone, and is primarily used on the back and legs. Percussion sounds and body movements begin slowly and softly, building up to a crescendo and stopping almost abruptly, with a slightly reducing finish that is shorter than the introduction.

1 Keeping the fingers and thumb tightly closed, soften and fold the fingers towards your palm, keeping the thumb straight and in contact with the index finger.

CAUTION

Cupping should make a hollow dull sound, not a slapping sound, as each cupped hand strikes the skin. If you make a slapping sound or leave red finger-marks on the skin, you are probably holding your hands too open and flat – adjust the position and try again.

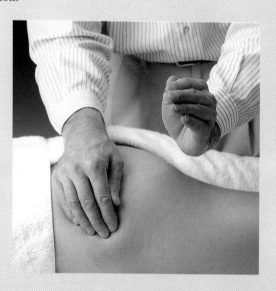

2 Turn your hand palm down. Lift one hand about two inches above the body surface, keeping the cupped hand positions. Now begin by dropping one hand and alternately lifting the other.

Hacking

Hacking stimulates the body's blood supply, along with the tissues and fibres.

1 Holding your hands straight, place them on the body surface with palms parallel approximately two inches apart. Relax your shoulders and let the elbows drop, losing the rigidity in the hands, yet maintaining strength.

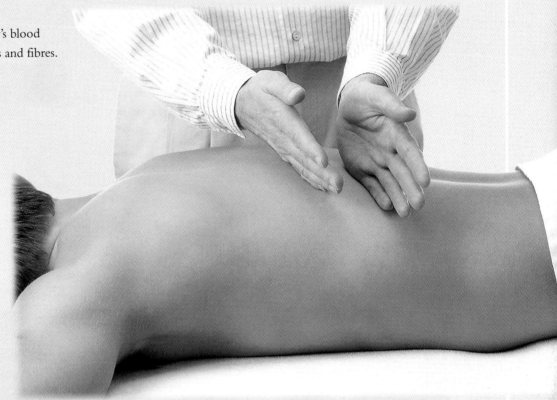

2 Pull back your right hand towards your body and with a flicking motion of the wrist, strike the skin with the lateral side of your hand in a 'chopping' action.

3 Now repeat using alternating hands. With practice, you will establish the pattern of hacking with ease and harmony, your fingers vibrating against one another as they strike the surface of the skin.

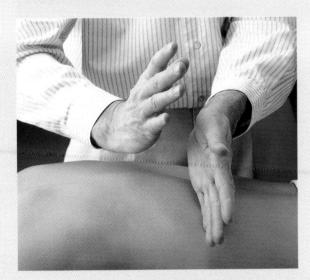

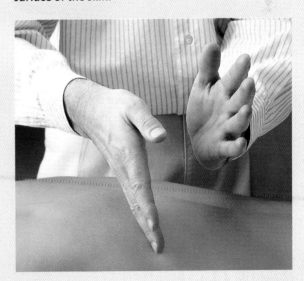

Vibration

The strong beating sound is performed on the large-muscled, well-padded areas of the body, for example the buttocks and thighs. The more powerful contact penetrates deep, stimulating the muscle fibres and layers.

You will need to drop your body and hence your body weight to get behind this movement, but remember that with all these percussion moves the action is generated from the wrist.

CAUTION

Take care not to strike any bony areas, however, as you may hurt both yourself and your partner, and you could jar the skeleton.

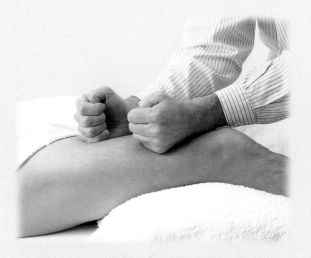

1 Hold your hands parallel and roll your fingers into a loose fist, placing the thumbs on top.

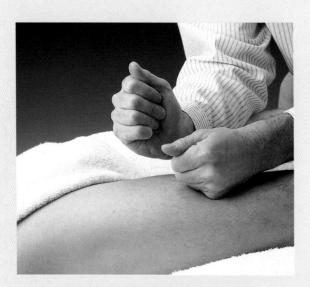

2 Now place both fists gently on the area to be pummelled – try starting with the upper thigh. Draw back the right wrist, releasing contact with the body, and then with a downward motion strike the body surface.

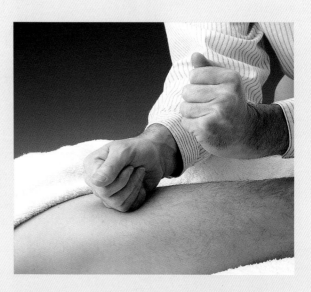

3 Continue by alternating the right and left hands to create a striking rhythm.

CAUTION

Buttocks are often an untouched area, and you may find that a lot of stress and tension are stored here. Begin lightly, and check the pressure throughout to avoid pain and discomfort to your partner.

Tapping or Tapotement

Tapping, also known as tapotement, has a finer 'pitter-patter' of heavy rainfall, stimulating the underlying surface of the skin. It can be safely applied to the face or other more delicate areas of the body. Tapping is relaxing but also stimulating, due to the trigger of reflex action, and is particularly pleasant when applied to the brow and face.

Rest your finger pads gently on the skin surface. Tap the small finger pad of each hand onto the skin surface, lifting the other digit pads. As you release the fifth zone pad, place the fourth zone finger pad. Repeat these finger actions, placing the third pad as you lift the fourth, the index finger pad as you lift the third, and finally the thumb as you lift the index

finger. At first you may find it helpful to turn your hand outward, almost palm up, then roll your wrists inwards as each finger pad in turn makes contact with the skin. Lift your hand and repeat. Now try to do the same fingertip movements one digit at a time without rolling, keeping the back of your hand pointing up and the fingers pointing down. You may find it easier to begin with your index finger and not use your thumb. Increase your finger speed, but keep it light!

Tapotement can also been done as a self-massage therapy for headache and tension in the head, face and face area, such as is caused by too much close work or staring at a computer screen.

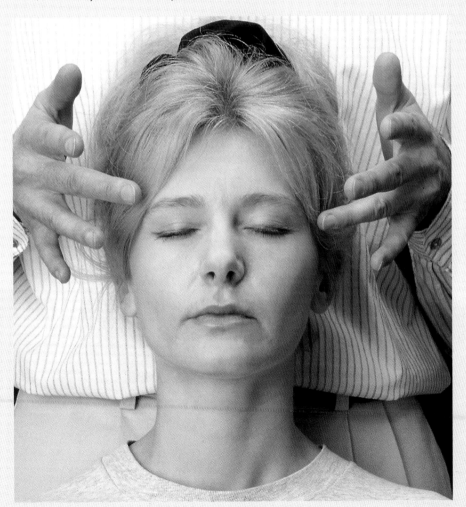

CAUTION
When tapping the face, avoid the area around the eye where skin is soft, thin and delicate.

Gentle tapping is very effective on sensitive areas such as the brow or face. The gentle rhythmic movements of the fingertips stimulate the tissue just below the skin.

Developing
Further Techniques

'Thumbing' involves applying pressure through the thumbs and moving them towards each other in a circular motion.

Further techniques can be incorporated into the movement following effleurage.

Fanning

Fanning combines effleurage with stretching and friction. It is effective over larger expanses of body tissues – along the back, for example, or the length of the leg (breaking contact at the back of the knee and the knee cap). Use steady, repetitive effleurage hand positions, modified by applying pressure with your fingers, held slightly relaxed and apart, slowly pushing the skin beneath in a gliding movement. Alternate the hands, keeping one hand in contact with the skin and as you lift the other hand for the retreating movement. With practice, you will find yourself applying massage in a moving meditation.

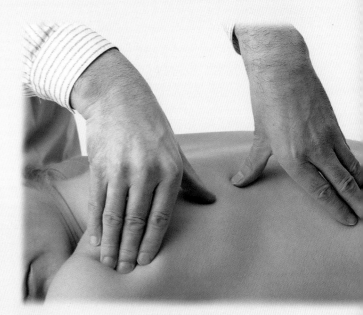

Thumbing

Thumbing can be used on localised sites where disharmony is present, indicated by a redness when effleurage is applied.

With open hands, depress your thumbs so that a slight indentation is made on the surface of the skin. Glide your thumbs toward each other with a small circular movement, then reverse the movement and repeat as necessary.

Alternate thumb pressure, rotating and pushing for deeper penetration of muscle fibres, can be beneficial to stressed, tension-stored areas of the skin. It is mainly applied to the upper back and calf muscles.

Fanning involves holding your fingers apart and gently stroking your partner in a soothing motion.

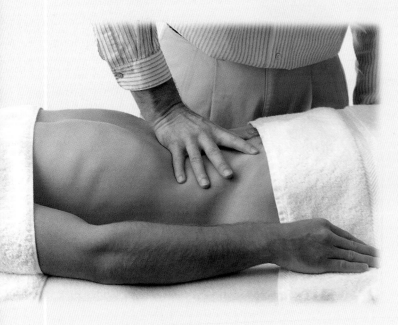

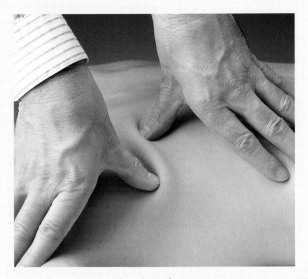

When effleurage causes redness this is often an indication of disharmony, which can be relieved by thumbing on specific spots.

Jostling

Jostling assists the relaxation of the muscle and encourages the body to let go of tension.

Grasp the muscle at the point of origin and shake gently, working your way up to the point of insertion.

Where there is extreme tension, jostling can be used to coax the muscles into letting go.

Standing at the side of your partner, trace the shape of the scapula from below the shoulder blade, moving up toward the shoulder for increased stimulation and circulation into and under the skeletal structure; then, standing at the head, thumb the shoulders from the top of the shoulder muscle areas, where tension is most likely to be stored.

For the back of the calves, trace from above the achilles area toward the back of knee (but do not press onto this area of soft tissue), using thumb rotation and depression in an upward movement towards the heart. Trace three lines, one central, one medial and one lateral. The latter two traces glide to the end of the muscle before the back of knee to aid venous flow and elimination of toxins from muscle fibres.

Fisting

As the name implies, the fist is used to apply pressure from the back of your hand.

With the fingers cupped into the palms and pointing towards you, bend the wrists and roll the knuckles onto the surface of the skin, applying pressure as you do so. Use a long fisting stroke down the centre of the back, 4cm either side of the spinal column, for stretch, and short circular deep movements into fatty areas, for example the buttocks, to release stored tension.

Instead of the flat of the hand, fisting uses the back of a clenched hand for applying deep pressure into fatty areas.

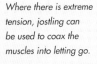

Storing Oils

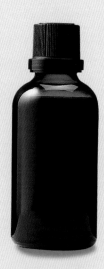

Keep oils in a cool, dark place. Small coloured glass bottles are ideal for storage.

Base oils should be kept in containers with airtight lids, and essential oils should be stored in dark glass containers as the chemical constituents can cause plastic to melt. Oils are volatile, so storing in direct sunlight should be avoided, while hot steamy conditions can cause the oil to go rancid.

If stored at too low a temperature, and sometimes when stored in a domestic refrigerator, oils can thicken. If this happens, simply leave the oils at room temperature before application, and they will return to liquid form.

Though you will find the oil will seem thicker and of a different consistency and absorptiont, it is safe to use base oils from the refrigerator. Warm the oil in your hands before applying.

Secure the lid of the container, as base oils will oxidise and essential oil will evaporate easily.

Make a note of the purchase date, or better still of the 'use by' date if there is one, because oils have a limited shelf life. The freshness of most base oils can easily be recognised – simply trust your senses as you

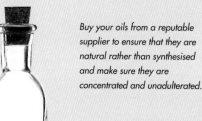

FRANKINCENSE

would in the kitchen when using cooking oils. If the appearance is dull, dark or cloudy, or if the smell is rancid or sour, do not use it.

Most citrus oils have a shelf life of six months, and some heavier essential oils, such as myrhh and frankincense last for up to two years. Because of the possibility of adulteration, it is important to ensure you buy oils from a reputable supplier.

Buy your oils from a reputable supplier to ensure that they are natural rather than synthesised and make sure they are concentrated and unadulterated.

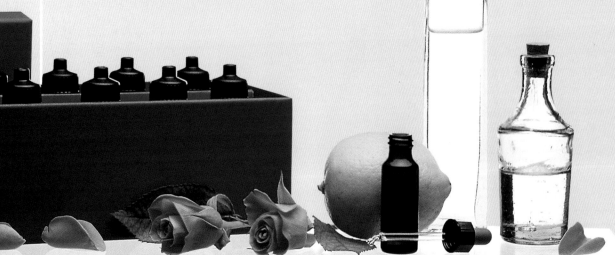

CARRIER OILS

Essential oils dissolve in fats, oils and pure alcohol. They do not dissolve in water, and so cannot be diluted except by adding base oil. Use vegetable-based oils, NOT mineral – sweet almond oil is recommended. Baby oils are not easily absorbed, and may contain benzol (petrol). Vitamin E or wheatgerm oil can be added to prolong shelf life, but large quantities of base oil will go rancid if not used up quickly, even with these oils added.

SAFETY

Keep the oils out of the reach of children. It is advisable to store oils in high, locked cabinets, as with medicine. If children ingest any oil, give them dry bread and milk to absorb it, and take them to your general practitioner should vomiting or diarrhoea follow. If a large amount of oil or essential oil has been taken, contact the Accident & Emergency Department of your local hospital for treatment and advice.

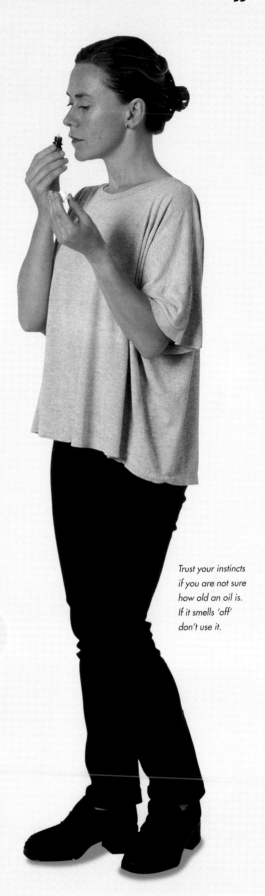

Trust your instincts if you are not sure how old an oil is. If it smells 'off' don't use it.

CAUTION

Oils are flammable – store them away from naked flames, and do not store next to the boiler or cooker.

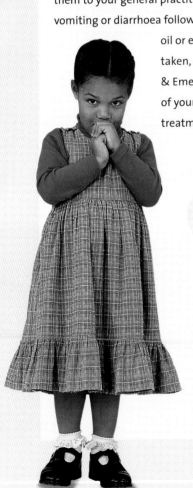

Children are often attracted by the lovely smells of essential oils, so make sure you store oils safely out of their reach.

Self-Massage

Many of us today choose to live alone – but do not think that massage is not for you, or that you will not benefit or be able to enjoy the positive effects of massage. You will be amazed how many parts of your own body you can reach, and how self-massage will increase your confidence – not to mention boost your immune system.

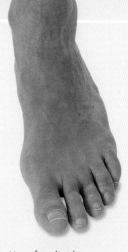

Most of us already massage aching feet effectively. It is a natural impulse.

FOOT CARE

Feet – they hold you up all day, relentlessly abused by shoes, pressures and stresses of everyday life. How often do you thank them?

The feet are to the body as foundations are to a house. If the foundations are not well taken care of, the walls of the house will eventually crack and further problems will follow. With your feet, if your arches are not functioning as shock absorbers, lower back pain and stress headaches may well present themselves. Pay attention to any dry skin – if left unattended, it may develop into cracks and sore wounds, open to infection. Cold feet, indicating poor circulation, can lead to cramp and/or chilblains.

If you don't have time to massage your feet, visualise them in a pool of healing blue-green water that is easing all your stiffness away. If time permits, do this visualisation as well as the foot massage.

FOOT MASSAGE

If today has been 'one of those days', try this short self-foot-massage to help you regain your well-being.

1 Remove all footwear where appropriate – stockinged feet are okay. Sit comfortably, perhaps with your favourite music playing softly in the background.

2 Feel your thighs with an open hand to each leg. Depress the flesh using a slight squeezing action between thumb and fingers, working your way from your thighs to your knees. Repeat several times, feeling tension release as you gently squeeze away aches caused by pressure and stress. Finish by 'brushing off' with a sweeping, gliding motion in the same direction.

> **FEET**
> See also the section on foot massage as part of a whole body massage.

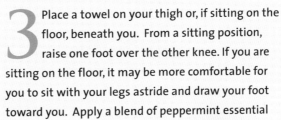

3 Place a towel on your thigh or, if sitting on the floor, beneath you. From a sitting position, raise one foot over the other knee. If you are sitting on the floor, it may be more comfortable for you to sit with your legs astride and draw your foot toward you. Apply a blend of peppermint essential oil, either with sweet almond oil or with cocoa butter if you have really dry skin. If you prefer, use talcum powder or leave on your socks or tights.

4 Hold your foot firmly, and with both hands easing out from the centre to the outer edges begin to massage your sole. You will find it easiest to apply pressure with your thumbs. Give the foot a good stretch.

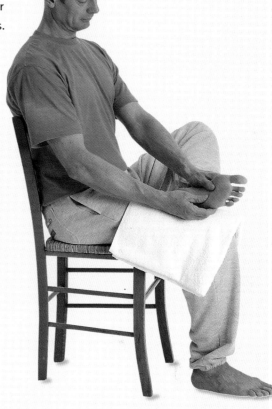

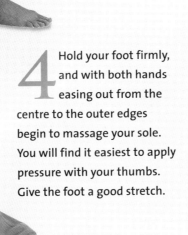

5 Massage around your ankles with circular motions. Gently rotate the ankle clockwise two or three times, then repeat anticlockwise.

6 Using your thumbs, massage with gentle pressure toward the toes, lightly trace the natural crevice between the toe phalanges, then move from your toes towards your ankles to drain the lymphatic tissue.

7 Hold your foot for a moment and say 'thank you' to yourself for this reward and 'thank you' to your feet for holding you up all day.

Whole Body Massage

It is possible to give yourself a whole body massage. You will need a firm, straight-backed chair. Take the time to create the right atmosphere with music, lighting and candles, and choose a time when you are sure that you will not be interrupted.

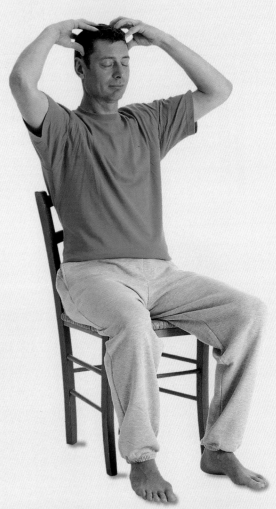

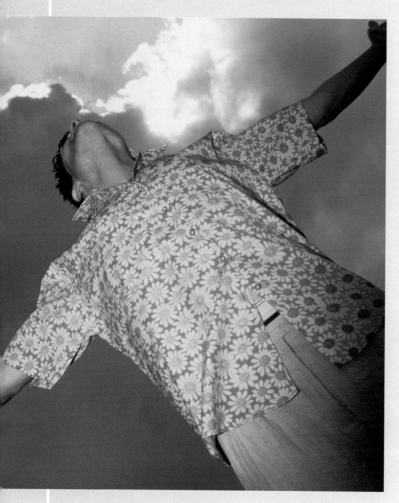

Giving yourself a whole body massage can be a very liberating and exhilarating experience.

1 Gently caress your scalp with your fingertips – fingers on top, thumbs pointing downwards. Circle your thumbs, and as they rotate you will find that your fingertips join in. Use this motion all over your crown, then lower your fingertips behind your head, allowing your thumbs to drop down into the nape of your neck, and rotate your fingers in larger circles. Next, very gently and without exerting pressure on the soft tissues and structure of your neck, take your palms either side of your neck with fingertips facing behind, and rotate in a minute circular motion.

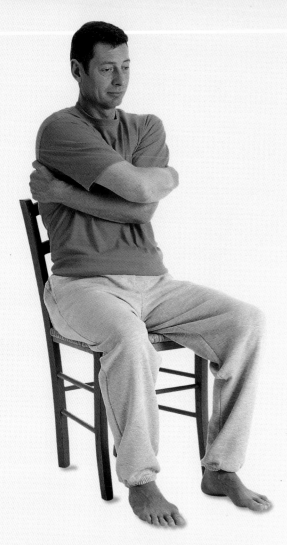

4 Open the palm of your left hand, relax, and now with your right thumb gently and softly rotate over the pads of your left palm. Supporting the fingers with the right hand, gently massage the three phalanges of each digit, including the thumb. Give a gentle pull on each finger. Change hands and repeat the massage to the right hand. Use a slight pulling action to stimulate and invigorate blood flow.

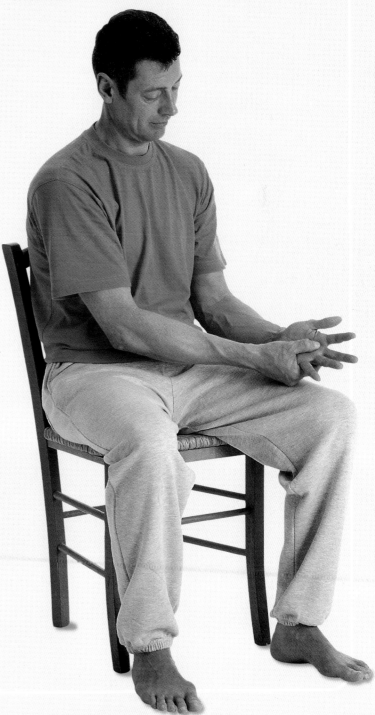

2 Moving on to your shoulders, following the contours of your body from your neck outward, press more firmly with the fingertips, still with a minute circular motion. Squeeze and pinch across your shoulders. Now cross your arms and embrace yourself – give yourself a squeeze and a hug, you deserve to be loved.

3 Squeeze your shoulders, moving down the tops of your arms. Repeat this several times, feeling the tension and pain held in your muscles releasing. Continue down the arm to your wrist with a grasping motion, hold, then allow your palm to slide off. With your thumbs, you can gently circle the left elbow, cupped In your right hand for support. Repeat with your right elbow cupped in your left hand.

5 With your finger pads, 'play the piano' on your shoulder. It may be most comfortable to cross your hands to the opposite shoulder, cupping your elbow in your hand for support and extra lift. Now patter your fingertips up and down and all around your scalp, even gently across your brow. This will stimulate the brain so that it is clearer, brighter and ready for action.

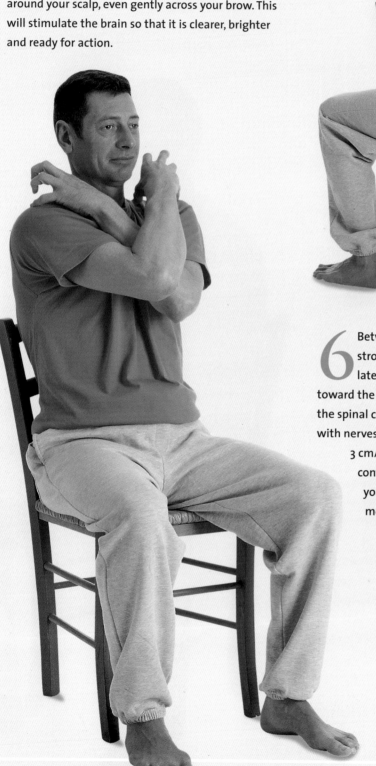

6 Between the last two steps, if you have time, stroke your back, placing the thumbs on your lateral sides and the fingertips pointing toward the spinal column. Avoid direct contact with the spinal column as this area has intricate disc space with nerves attached, but you are quite safe 3 cm/1¼ in either side. As your hands fall to the contour of your back in the lumbar region, you will be able to make larger circular movements with your palms.

7 With open hands, thumb inward and fingers outward, jostle and press your thighs, lifting, squeezing and almost pinching, but taking care not to bruise your skin. Work your way down toward your knees, and repeat three times.

9 With your right hand, cup the large calf muscle of your left leg, squeezing with the open V of the hand. Stroke the shin bone, and hold your foot for a moment, massaging gently and not forgetting the toes. Release the leg and give the calves a stretch by pushing the heel downward and releasing, then pointing your toes and releasing. Finally, rotate your ankle and repeat to right leg.

GROUNDING

When you finish, or at any time, try applying tapotement to your scalp, stimulating the brain receptors. Stand up and brush yourself down with long strokes to ground yourself, ready to take on the world again.

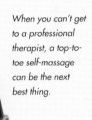

When you can't get to a professional therapist, a top-to-toe self-massage can be the next best thing.

8 Now hold your knees in the palms of your hands, gently massaging them with your fingers in circular movements from below the knee cap, working outward around the natural shape to the top of the knee and back down on the inside, keeping the touch light. If it is appropriate and you are physically able to do so, try lifting the knees one at a time back toward your body, supported by your hands, to stretch the thigh muscles.

Massage at **Work**

Instead of stopping for a coffee break, use the time instead to apply some massage either to yourself or to a colleague – or ask a colleague to massage you. Even just a five-minute shoulder rub will ease tension and set you up for the rest of the day.

Hectic schedules mean we rush around with our muscles tense and our breathing shallow, restricting our natural energy flows.

Eating cakes during the working day upsets the balance of your blood sugar levels.

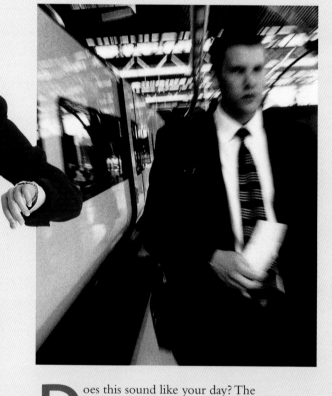

Heavy bags and shoes with high heels pull the body out of alignment, leading to aching muscles and tension in the body.

Does this sound like your day? The commuting journey to the office was hectic and crowded. There was so much traffic on the road you were worried you would miss your train. There was no buffet car, so you had no breakfast, and although you had a healthy salad-filled sandwich for lunch, you followed it with a sticky bun and coffee, upsetting the balance of your blood sugar levels. You have had deadlines to keep and people to meet – it's all smiles and endless conversation. You know you would benefit from a massage, but you cannot spare the time to leave the office.

So what is the answer? Use your lunchtime to give yourself a massage. It is not necessary to undress – simply remove your jacket. Set the scene by closing the office door and letting Reception know that you are at lunch and will not be taking any calls. Put on a CD of restful melodies – not your favourite rock band – or better still that relaxation tape you were drawn to but have not really had the opportunity to listen to yet. Dim the lights and, if possible, draw the blinds, closing off the outside world, and simply follow the instructions for the whole body massage.

With work-place massage, join a colleague if possible. Take it in turns to give each other a back massage, leaning forward on the desk from your chair. It is not necessary to remove clothing, but you may prefer to remove your jackets and heavy pullovers. If it feels good, do it. Your colleague just became your friend!

Tension headaches caused by close work can be relieved by applying gentle pressure to the scalp or tapotement to the face.

Even just a few minutes' time out and a gentle shoulder massage from a colleague will ease tension and refresh you.

Sensual Massage

Sharing a sensual massage is rewarding and beneficial to both parties. Massage between two people is connecting and sharing, giving and taking. The feeling of well-being and of being cared for is made more sensual by keeping the massage strokes lighter and the contact longer.

Don't forget areas such as your elbows, both outer and inner, and your ears, which are so often not touched. When massaging the neck, which for many holds a great deal of tension, lengthen the strokes from the shoulders sensuously, taking your hands past the neck to the ears, head and side of the face.

Sensuality requires trust. If you can free yourself of life's restricting inhibitions you will be able to give and receive more sensual massage. You will both need to release stored tensions and insecurities, so take it in turn to be massaged. Communicate during the massage, letting your partner know when the touch applied feels good or if it is too heavy. Strokes applied too deeply may cause pain and discomfort, but strokes applied too lightly may lead the massaged person to fall asleep. The key is to vary the strokes and to find out what your partner likes best.

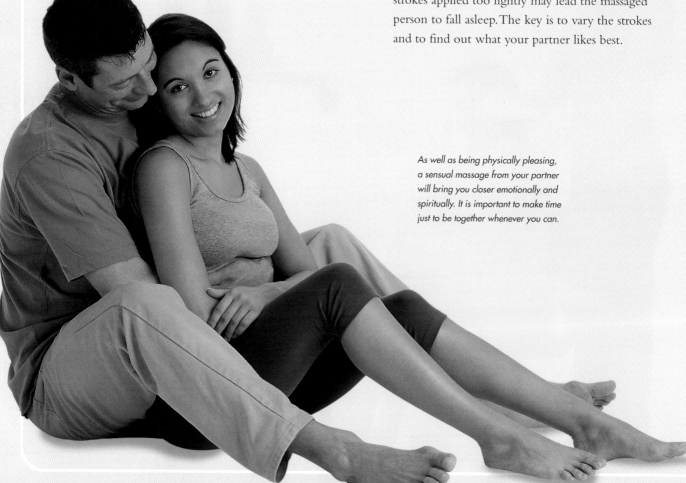

As well as being physically pleasing, a sensual massage from your partner will bring you closer emotionally and spiritually. It is important to make time just to be together whenever you can.

1 Set the scene. Make sure that your room is warm. Wear minimal clothing. Have towels and oil to hand. Put on soft music, dim the lights and perhaps scatter some rose petals.

2 With your partner lying on their front, position yourself at your partner's head. Effleurage on either side of the spine (not on the spine itself), stroking the skin as you apply the oil all over their back. Start at the nape of neck and move your hands towards the buttocks close to the spine on the way down and to the sides of the body on the way back up. Repeat three times. Now extend this movement to include the buttock cheeks on the way down and the shoulders and top of the arms on the way back. Repeat three times. Squeezing the buttocks releases stored tension.

3 Massage your partner's head with firm but gentle circular strokes, as you would when shampooing your hair. Stroke the hair and head to finish this area. Rubbing the skull quite firmly relieves tension; a soothing stroke can lift depression. Gathering and tugging the hair stimulates the circulation, but remember to keep it gentle.

4 Move on to your partner's legs. Stroke up the back of the legs, one hand following the other from heels to buttocks and gliding down again, tracing the outer contours of the leg. Gently stroke the areas behind the knees. Feather your hand strokes from thigh to heel and then hold the heel.

5 Invite your partner to turn over to lie on their back.

6 Massage their face and scalp with gentle circular movements. Circle their temples and beneath their cheek bones to release stress. Stroke from the shoulder line gently along their neck to their chin. In a rolling action, gently pinch the chin between your finger and thumb.

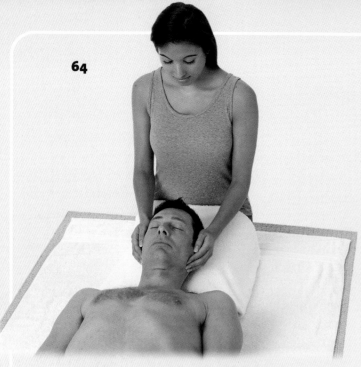

10 Massage your partner's torso with the back of your hands; stroke gently as you trace the outer contours of the trunk. Take your hand to your partner's shoulder and trace the shoulder-line to the side of their neck, applying gentle pressure in the neck region. Continue with small circles tracing the contours of your partner's chest or breasts. Take your index fingers to the end of this area down the centre of the trunk and walk your fingers softly and gently from beneath the breast bone to the navel.

11 Continue the massage into the thigh region. If you can reach, stand at your partner's feet and massage one leg in each hand. Form open 'V' with each hand and and push the skin upward in the direction of your partner's head. Glide your hand down the outer contours of the leg. If you cannot reach to do this, massage one leg from side of your partner's body then move round and repeat on the other leg. Alternatively, you could place their lower leg on your shoulders as you massage their thighs, but remember to return their legs gently to the table before massaging the lower leg.

7 Now massage your partner's ear lobes. Gently squeezing between your forefinger and thumb, work your way up and down the outer part of the ears and then down the inside of the ears three times. Cup your hands over the ears, palms flattened and with very light pressure move your hands up and down and then circle your hands for heightened sensuality. Gently pull the ears up and down. If you're feeling playful, flick the ear lobes – not too hard or too often as this causes a red hot tingly sensation as energy rushes down through the whole body. The Chinese art of acupressure maps over two hundred points corresponding to the body on the small surface of your ear!

8 Move to your partner's side. First apply oil with effleurage strokes to their torso and arms. Trace the contours of your partner's inner arm. The areas on the outer sides of trunk and inner arms are rarely touched and are thin skinned therefore very sensitive. Keep your strokes very full in length from the shoulder down the arm. Keep contact until reaching the fingertips. Repeat four times.

9 Gently stroke the inner crease of your partner's elbow and touch gently the wrist crease and the palm of your partner's hands with your fingertips. The senses are now heightened and this can become quite ticklish as well as sensual.

12 Effleurage their thighs, picking up muscle using hand in 'V' shape. Standing at your partner's side, move one hand in front of the other along their leg in an open-handed V. Circle each knee cap, tracing it between your thumb and forefinger. Caress the backs of the knees with your fingertips.

13 Continue down the leg, maintaining contact until reach the tips of the toes. Hold the feet in your hands, standing by the feet facing your partner's head. Cup the feet well and cradle them with your hands. You could rest their feet on your lap or knee. With a little more firmness apply thumb rotations from the heel up the soles of your partner's feet; stroke your hand off by gliding back down and flicking off at their heels. You can grasp their ankles, holding the feet behind their heels. Then lean forward and request your turn!

Before you Start

It is important to create the right atmosphere for massage. It is frustrating for both parties if the mood is broken by interruptions or if the patient cannot get comfortable enough to relax and enjoy the treatment. Make sure everything you need is to hand before you begin.

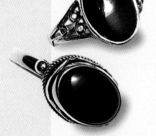

Rings might cause irritation, so remove them before massage.

SETTING THE SCENE

Allow sufficient time. If you allow only ten minutes because you are massaging 'only' your hand, you will find that you have become absorbed and time just sails on by.

Set the scene with gentle music, low lighting, and a notice for 'no interruptions'.

Remove jewellery.

Slow down for greater relaxation to both you and your partner, and greater control of movement and applied pressure.

Centre yourself at the beginning and throughout the massage.

Cover your massage partner with a towel, exposing only the area you are massaging.

Prepare the base oil. If you are adding essential oils, prepare your blend, checking any particular likes or dislikes, because smells have strong associations. Do not blend more than three oils because chemical reactions take place with the plants' properties.

Make sure you are both comfortable.

It is important to encourage your partner to feel comfortable. It is no good if, when you begin massaging, your partner feels the need to move a limb and is unable to do so freely.

Uncross the legs.

Check that you are both ready to begin.

Be calm. Relax. Centre yourself.

Pull back the towel gently and slowly, exposing only the body part to be massaged

Get connected: lay your hands gently for a moment and try not to break contact – leave one hand or fingertip on your partner's body whenever possible.

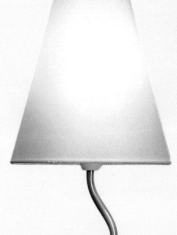

Select a level of lighting with which you are both comfortable. It needs to be soft but not gloomy.

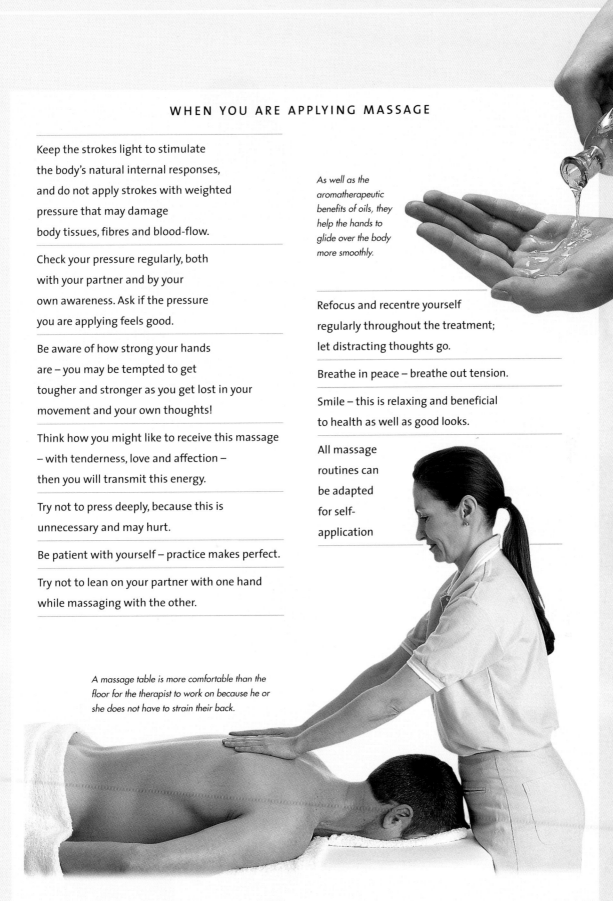

WHEN YOU ARE APPLYING MASSAGE

Keep the strokes light to stimulate
the body's natural internal responses,
and do not apply strokes with weighted
pressure that may damage
body tissues, fibres and blood-flow.

Check your pressure regularly, both
with your partner and by your
own awareness. Ask if the pressure
you are applying feels good.

Be aware of how strong your hands
are – you may be tempted to get
tougher and stronger as you get lost in your
movement and your own thoughts!

Think how you might like to receive this massage
– with tenderness, love and affection –
then you will transmit this energy.

Try not to press deeply, because this is
unnecessary and may hurt.

Be patient with yourself – practice makes perfect.

Try not to lean on your partner with one hand
while massaging with the other.

*As well as the
aromatherapeutic
benefits of oils, they
help the hands to
glide over the body
more smoothly.*

Refocus and recentre yourself
regularly throughout the treatment;
let distracting thoughts go.

Breathe in peace – breathe out tension.

Smile – this is relaxing and beneficial
to health as well as good looks.

All massage
routines can
be adapted
for self-
application

*A massage table is more comfortable than the
floor for the therapist to work on because he or
she does not have to strain their back.*

Face Massage

The face is very sensitive and while this means it is receptive to massage, it can also be difficult for a person to relax properly when their face is being touched. Trust needs to be built up between the partners if this effective massage is to be successful.

1 Put your hands together, spreading oil thinly and equally between your palms. Standing at the head position, very gently start applying oil to the skin with a stroking motion. Avoid the eye area (soft tissue around the eyes draws moisture toward the eyes). Stroke the forehead from the centre outward very gently with the fingertips, rounding the motion to finish at the hair line as you lift your hand clear to begin the movement again at the centre. Repeat six times.

2 Using the middle or ring fingers (to apply less body pressure), circle the temporal area six times.

3 Move the hands down adjacent to the middle-ear flap, feel for the dimple area and gently circle six times to relieve stress.

4 Spread your thumbs from the centre of the forehead out toward hairline. Repeat.

5 Very slowly and very gently, place the hands over the face, lifting the cupped palm over the eye area. Leave there for a few moments.

6 Lifting the heel of the hands, allow the fingers to smooth outward in a stroking motion, and hold the hands over the ears for a moment.

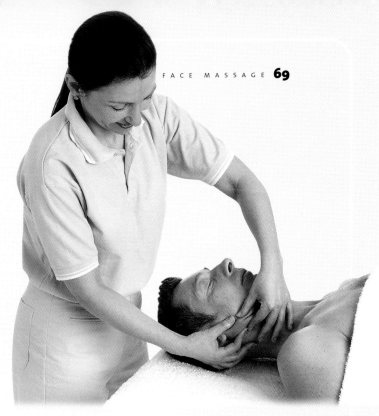

7 Feel along the cheek bone with gentle fingertips, depressing lightly in a pulling motion toward you to release stored tension.

8 Incorporate effleurage strokes from the shoulder lines along the neck to the chin line.

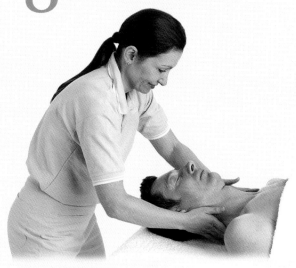

9 Finish the cheek area with a circular inward motion.

10 As you feel a little more confident, you can lightly and carefully depress around the eyes and the brow bones.

11 Stroke the nose with alternate middle fingers from between eyebrows downward and outward, gently stopping with a small circular pressure at the nose edge.

12 Place the fingertips gently together at the chin, moving the fingers outward and circling the end of the jaw line under the ears.

13 Begin at one side of jaw, with the thumb on the face side of the jaw and and the fingertips under the chin side. Gently roll your thumb and fingers in a pick-up and roll motion. Release and repeat as you work your way along the jaw to finish at the other ear.

14 Massage the ear lobes between thumb and fingers, and gently trace the outer ear.

15 Gently apply tapotement to the forehead with the fingertips in a rapid soft movement for stimulation.

16 Place the hands over the face again, pause and continue to finish by holding the ears gently.

Neck and Shoulder Massage

This can be added to the face massage, which feels more complete when it is continued into the neck and shoulders.

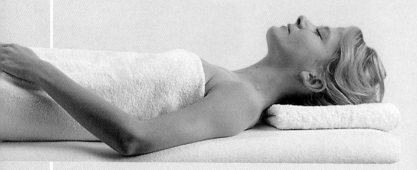

3 Gently, with the help of your forearm if you feel comfortable, or with a firm but gentle hand movement cupping the face, roll the right side of the neck, turning the head to face the left shoulder.

1 This massage is applied in the anterior position. Pull back the towel to show the collar bone area. Nudge the shoulders by a gentle rocking movement with hands placed on the shoulders laterally. Now nudge gently downward toward feet, lengthening the neck and dropping the shoulders.

2 Apply oil to your palm and rub your hands together. Oil your partner with effleurage stroking movements.

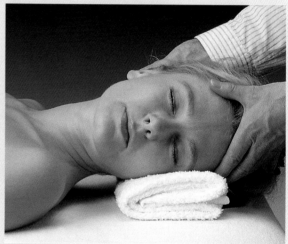

4 With a deep stroking movement, take your right hand from the shoulder, drawing and stroking toward the neck with the whole hand, releasing to fingers (two pads/phalanges) as you stroke up the side of the neck.

5 Allow your fingers to finish in the base of hairline. Repeat three times.

6 With two hands cupping, hold and guide the head back to the centre position, or you can use your forearm with practice.

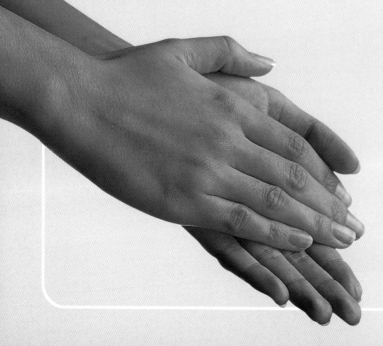

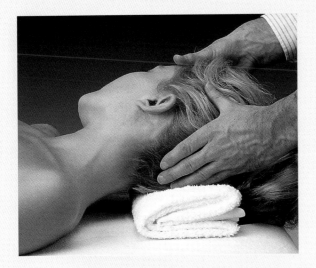

9 With a pull-back motion from the occipital area (base skull hairline), stretch the neck and head with the fingertips, once only. Run the fingers through the hair and massage the scalp with small circular movements, as if applying shampoo. Finish the scalp massage by gently teasing the hair through the fingers with a gentle pull/tug.

10 Place the hands gently on the shoulders with light pressure to end this massage. Hold the contact for a reassuring moment.

7 Repeat the massage, this time turning the head to face the right shoulder. Take your left hand from the shoulder, repeat the drawing stroking movement toward the neck, allowing the finger pads to stroke up the side of the neck, finishing in the hair-line. Repeat three times. Return the head to the centre again.

TIP
After turning the head to the side make sure that it is realigned properly with the spine before finishing the massage.

8 Take both hands in a large, slow, gentle yet firm move and stroke from the shoulders inward to the neck, then changing to finger-pad pressure effleurage the neck, gliding gently up the neck to the hair-line. Gently depress at the hair-line to finish this move.

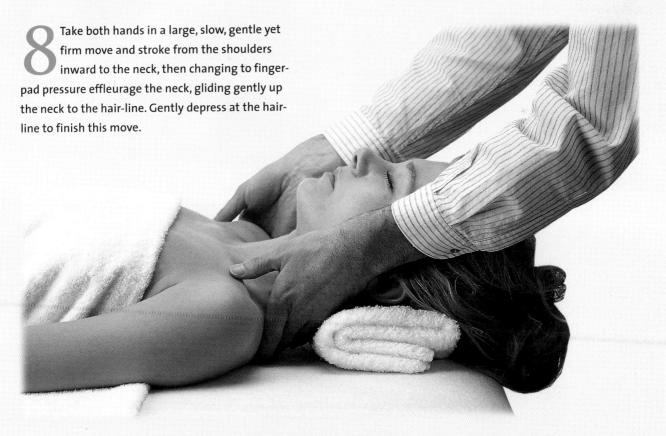

Abdomen Massage

Be gentle with the abdomen because it is a very sensitive area. Too much pressure can be painful and potentially damaging.

1 Ensure your partner is comfortable, warm and modestly covered in towels. Remove the towel carefully not to expose the chest/breast area. Connect by cupping the hands over the *hara* (just below the navel); feel the energy.

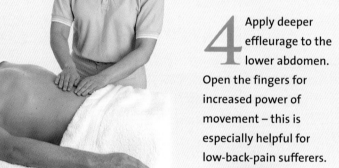

2 Apply the massage oil with effleurage in gentle circles, gradually increasing in size to trace the rib cage.

3 Knead with alternate hands, keeping the V of the hand quite open, moving up and down the abdomen and outer (lateral) sides of the body.

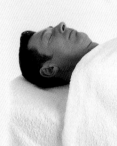

4 Apply deeper effleurage to the lower abdomen. Open the fingers for increased power of movement – this is especially helpful for low-back-pain sufferers.

5 Apply finger drainage, tracing the ribs and below the rib cage with thumbs from the sternum outward.

CAUTION
Check for any contra-indications before applying this massage. This massage is applied in the supine position (lying on the back).

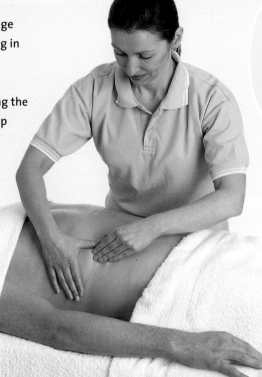

6 With finger pads, one hand on the other to exert controlled pressure, apply small circles, tracing the colon.

7 Trace circles around the abdomen with alternate hands, applying light pressure. Repeat three to four circles.

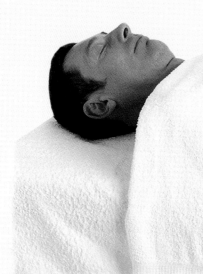

8 With fingertips facing the head, fan out your hands under the sides of the rib cage and with a lifting movement from under the back glide back up until the fingers meet over the abdomen. Repeat three times.

9 Circle the abdomen with one hand or alternate two hands, circling the abdomen three times.

10 Cup the hands and hold for a moment over the *hara* navel area to centre energy and to finish. Cover with towel. Cup hands again over *hara* and hold until energy gathers.

CAUTION

Use a light touch – remember that the abdomen is to be touched gently because the organs are very vulnerable.

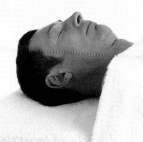

Arm Massage

Thorough effleurage of the arms not only relaxes the arms and shoulders but also helps to stimulate the lymphatic draining system.

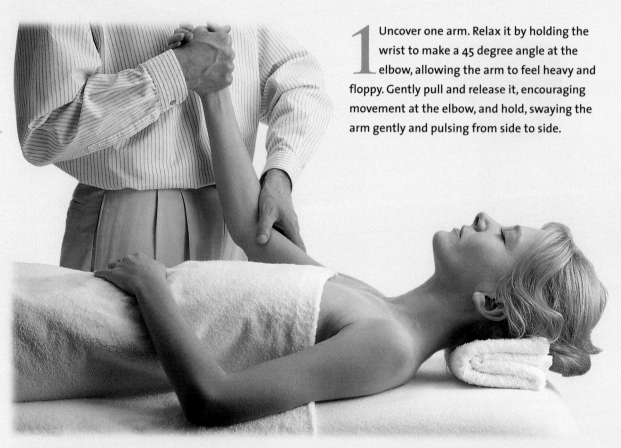

1 Uncover one arm. Relax it by holding the wrist to make a 45 degree angle at the elbow, allowing the arm to feel heavy and floppy. Gently pull and release it, encouraging movement at the elbow, and hold, swaying the arm gently and pulsing from side to side.

2 Lower the arm and apply oil by effleurage movements along the arm, firstly from the wrist crease to the elbow six times, and then from the elbow to the shoulder expanse six times.

3 Anchor the arm gently at the wrist with your free hand, and effleurage with a gliding movement from the wrist to the shoulder, gliding back to the wrist.

4 Span the fingers around the shoulder and trace with your thumb to ease around the joint. Smooth and effleurage the shoulder region.

TIP
Make sure you keep the rest of the body covered while massaging the arms, or your partner may get cold.

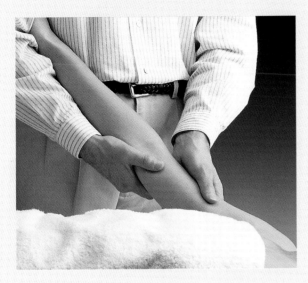

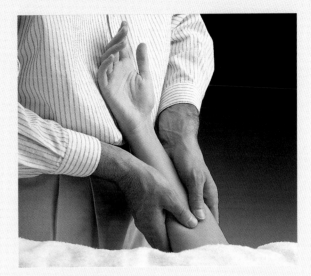

5 Repeat the movement from the wrist crease with the V of the hand in a pulsing and pumping action up the arm to the shoulder. Lift off applied pressure over the inside of the elbow crease, but trace around the elbow joint with finger and thumb.

6 Turn the arm over with the palm upward and gently drain the inner forearm. Your partner's fingers may spontaneously respond with a curling to opening movement as you apply petrissage between your finger and thumb. You can also bend the arm at the elbow with fingers pointing upward and trace down the forearm, squeezing gently.

7 Repeat this drainage to the upper arm, tracing the skeletal and muscle contour to assist lymphatic drainage.

8 Effleurage repeatedly the upper and lower arm, bringing in the whole length of the arm for completeness.

9 Finish with a long, slow, palm-hand movement, gliding up the arm and sliding slowly back to the wrist (at this point you can apply a gentle stretch with one hand at the wrist crease, while massaging with the other).

Hand Massage

This massage can follow the arm massage, or be applied on its own if time is short.

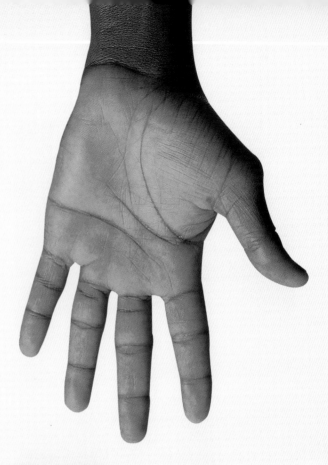

1 Turn the hand over, placing the arm comfortably on the couch. Massage the back of the hand, gently applying oil.

2 Trace the tendons of the hand with the thumbs by softly continuing the line between each finger toward the wrist. Turn the hand over, palm up.

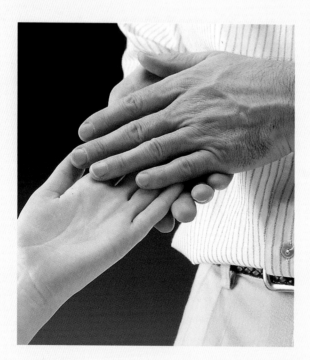

3 Massage the palm of the hand using the heel of your hand. Complete the movement by gently sweeping your hand to the fingertips.

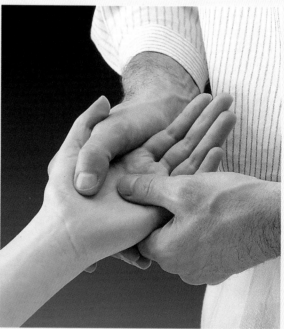

4 Spread and stretch the hand (this looks painful, but is not!) as you use your thumbs to trace and circle petrissage movements. When you feel more confident, open the hand further by hooking your little fingers under the thumb and fifth digit and massaging with your thumbs.

5 Turn the hand over, and holding the tip of each finger in turn use a rotate and pull-off friction from the knuckle to the tip to finish each finger.

6 Massage the back of the hand, either holding the hand in both your hands or holding the palm with one hand and massaging with other hand, smoothing and tracing from the knuckles to the wrist with a gentle circular thumb movement. Don't forget to trace the thumb crease too. Place the hand gently on the couch, palm down.

8 Cover slowly and gently with the towel. Walk round to the other side and repeat the procedure to the other arm.

7 Repeat effleurage from the wrist to the shoulder to give a complete feel to the massage, ending with a slow glide back to the hand and along the third digit, releasing the contact. Hold the hand for a moment as you place it comfortably back on the couch.

Leg Massage

Legs are well muscled and fleshy, so they benefit from strong, deep massage, including kneading and pummelling. It is important to work the joints as well.

1 Place a pillow or rolled towel under the knees to support the lower back if required. Fold back the towel to expose one leg, taking care to keep the other leg covered.

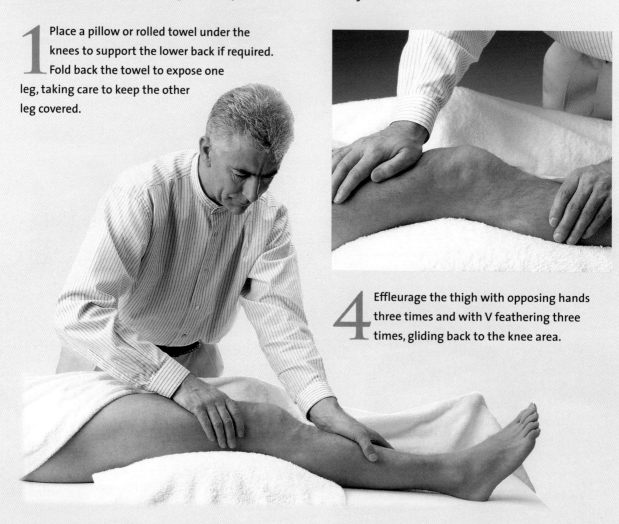

4 Effleurage the thigh with opposing hands three times and with V feathering three times, gliding back to the knee area.

2 Apply oil with effleurage strokes to the whole leg. Massage the front of the leg with effleurage, taking care not to press on the knee area.

3 From the foot upward, effleurage with the V of the hand, lifting the hands around the knee but tracing with fingers and thumb.

5 Trace around the knee-cap with the thumbs. Move the knee-cap gently from side to side with the thumbs.

6 Working from the foot toward the knee, it is possible to trace the shin with the thumbs along the skeleton (optional).

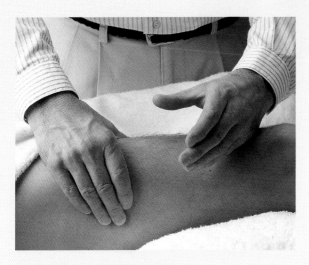
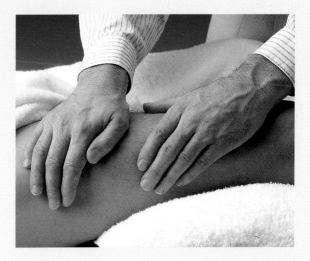

7 With open V of hands opposing, begin kneading the thigh, moving up and down the thigh six times.

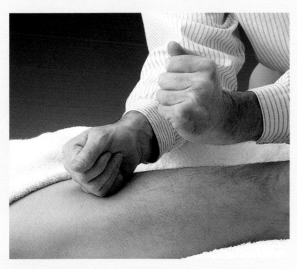

8 If required, perform pummelling with softly closed fists and cupping of percussion techniques to the upper thigh.

9 Apply the petrissage technique of thumb rolling. Be careful when squeezing the thinner skin and muscle fibres of the inner thigh as this area can pinch easily.

10 Return the leg to the flat position, supporting it, and check the position is comfortable before continuing.

11 Effleurage the complete leg at least three times, hand leading hand, gliding down the leg and stroking down the foot to complete the movement.

12 A gentle stretch can be performed by standing at the feet facing the head, cupping beneath the heel with one hand, and supporting and holding the foot with your other hand as you gently tug the foot toward your own body.

13 Effleurage the complete leg and glide over the foot to finish. At this point you can cover the leg with the towel, leaving the foot and ankle exposed for a foot massage.

14 If finishing here, hold the foot for a moment sandwiched between both hands, then cover the leg with the towel and move to the other side to repeat with the other leg.

Cupping the foot beneath the heel with one hand, support and hold the foot with the other.

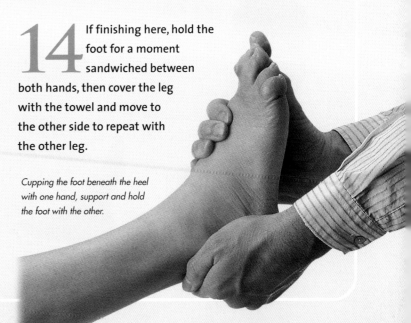

Foot Massage

When time is short a foot massage can be very beneficial. If your feet are in good spirits, then so are you! A version of this massage can also be done to yourself.

RELAXATION
Make the relaxation techniques slow and smooth for deep relaxation (or increase vigour for energy).

1 For a foot massage, your partner can be horizontal or in a semi-supine relaxed position. You can support and raise the feet by placing a rolled-up towel under the ankles toward the calf if required.

2 Uncover the right foot. Stand at the feet, facing the head. Greet the feet! – yes, say 'hello' and hold with your hands.

3 Relax the foot by cupping your hands on either side and gently rocking in a push-pull movement.

4 Relax the diaphragm by lightly but firmly pressing the thumb of your left hand over the solar plexus region – kidney 1, and with your right hand gently teasing the toes toward you in an up-and-over movement, working your way across whole line of the foot.

5 Free the ankle by gently rotating in the palms of your hands in a rocking push-pull movement.

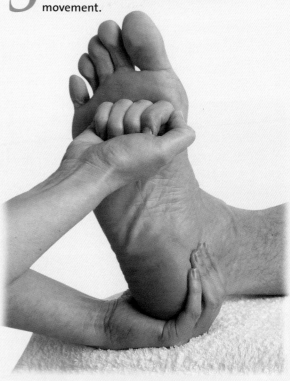

6 Apply oil between both your hands, and taking the foot in the left hand, work the heel of the right hand into the sole of the foot in a circular movement. Follow this with the fist kneading into the sole, gently but firmly.

7 The thumbs can be used to trace the instep, not so lightly as to tickle but not with your body weight behind the pressure applied, as this can affect the digestive system.

8 Trace the dorsal areas toward the toes between digits.

9 With a very small circular motion, take each toe individually and massage with your thumb dorsal area.

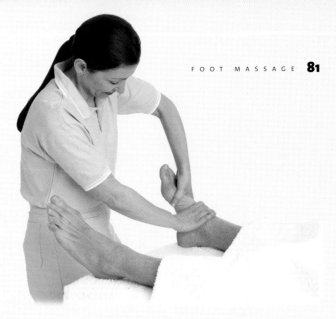

13 You can also use a wringing action along the spine of the foot.

14 With opposing hands, gently massage the dorsal from toes to ankle.

15 With the heel of your hands cupped around the heel of the foot, rotate circles, staying in the bony area of the heel.

16 Finish off with effleurage by gliding from ankle to toes with a pulling-off action at the end. Cover with the towel and hold the foot and leg for a moment before moving onto the other side. Repeat with the other foot.

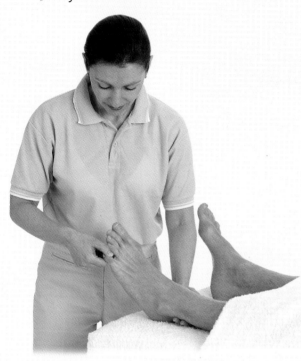

10 With fingers light but firm, gently rotate and stretch each toe with a pulling-off action to finish each digit.

11 Cupping the foot with the thumbs at midline, effleurage the sole, feathering outward.

12 Stretch the foot open by turning the thumbs outward and then relax, return the thumbs to midline, and pull the fingers toward you, stretching the dorsal gently.

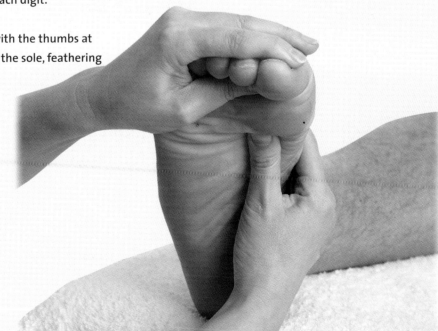

Calf, Thigh and **Buttock** Massage

When the front of the body is complete, ask your partner in a soft voice to turn over: 'Please turn over slowly and in your own time.'

1 This massage is applied in the posterior position. Make sure your partner is lying comfortably in the prone position, covered modestly with towels.

2 Uncover one leg. With oil, begin effleurage to the whole leg from toes to buttock.

3 Effleurage the lower leg and, with the V of the hands opposing, alternate rolling effleurage from the heel to behind the knee.

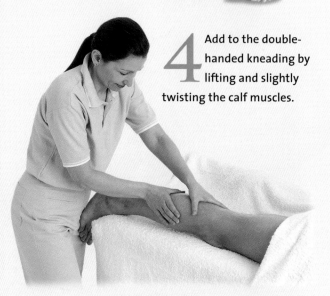

4 Add to the double-handed kneading by lifting and slightly twisting the calf muscles.

5 From the ankle, with alternate thumbs feather up the calf with hands in a V, fingers projecting out. Trace second and third imaginary lines behind the muscle either side of the first central line to cover first central, second lateral and third median.

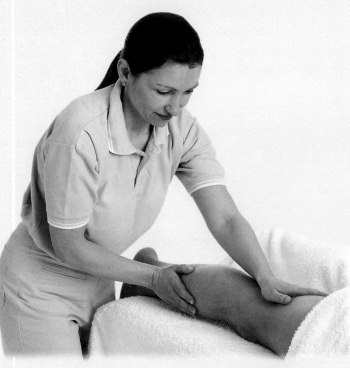

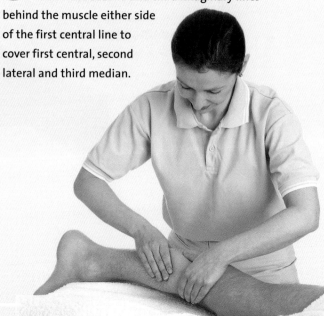

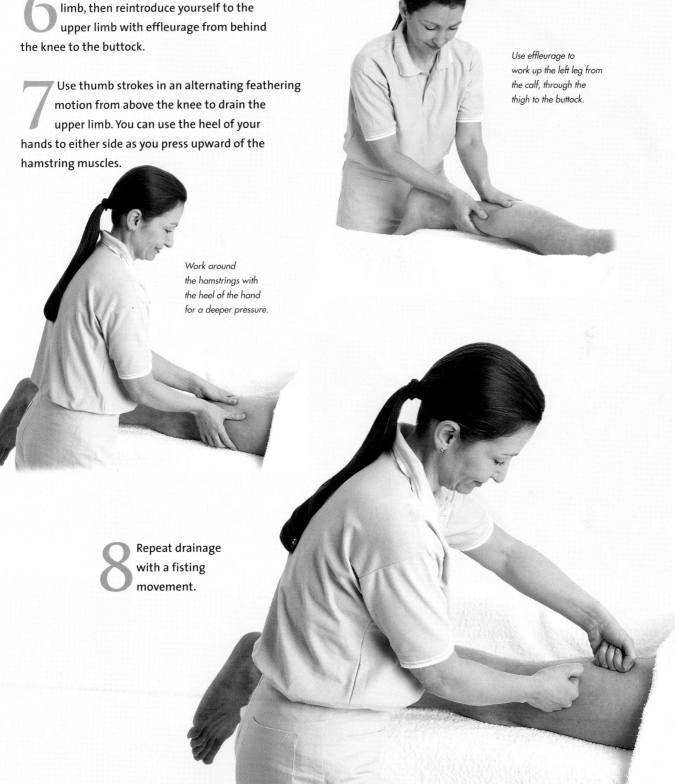

6 Repeat effleurage to soothe the lower limb, then reintroduce yourself to the upper limb with effleurage from behind the knee to the buttock.

Use effleurage to work up the left leg from the calf, through the thigh to the buttock.

7 Use thumb strokes in an alternating feathering motion from above the knee to drain the upper limb. You can use the heel of your hands to either side as you press upward of the hamstring muscles.

Work around the hamstrings with the heel of the hand for a deeper pressure.

8 Repeat drainage with a fisting movement.

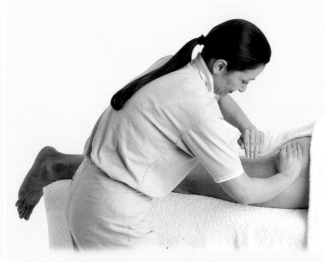

9 Try hands-cupped percussion movements over fatty areas of the thigh and into the buttocks (use the edge of your hand in a fist to chop or the flat edge of your hand to hack). Work on the large gluteus muscle of the buttock.

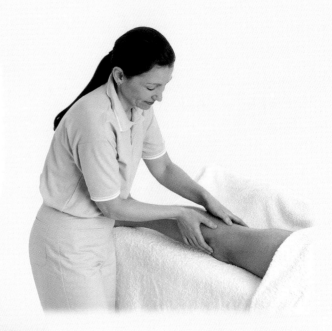

11 Gently circle the thumbs over the back of the knee area.

10 Effleurage the thigh area, gliding gently to the back of the knee.

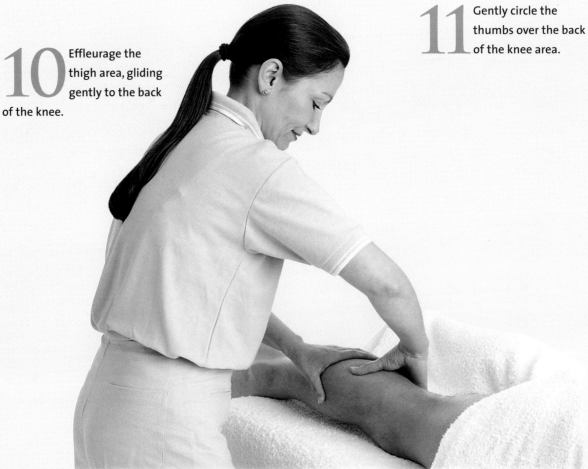

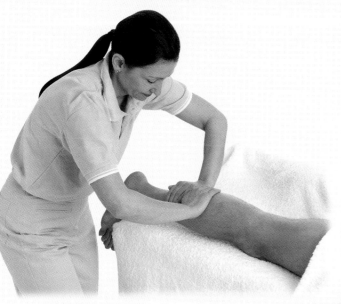

TIP
The buttocks often store up a lot
of stress, but they can also be very ticklish.
Use your judgement about how your
partner will react to this part
of the massage.

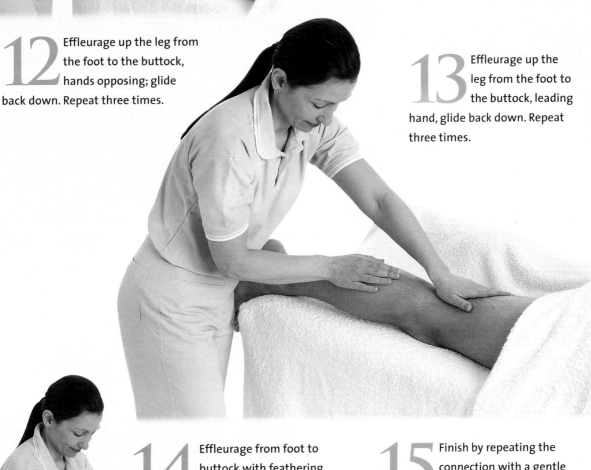

12 Effleurage up the leg from the foot to the buttock, hands opposing; glide back down. Repeat three times.

13 Effleurage up the leg from the foot to the buttock, leading hand, glide back down. Repeat three times.

14 Effleurage from foot to buttock with feathering movement, glide back down. Repeat three times and finish the stroke down the sole of the foot.

15 Finish by repeating the connection with a gentle stretch. Hold the ankle and leg for a moment.

16 Cover with the towel. Then repeat the sequence on the other leg.

Back Massage

A full back massage is often complemented with a head massage, although this is not essential. A combination of techniques can be used for massaging the back.

1 Check that your partner is warm, comfortable and modestly covered with towels. Connect with your partner. From the head, nudge the shoulders gently with a rocking motion.

2 From the side, stretch the back from the middle using both hands held apart – at the finish of each stretch, hold for a moment.

3 Remove towel. If you are confident, you can cross your arms diagonally, placing one hand on the shoulder and the other on the buttock, and stretch the back. Repeat stretch from the other shoulder to the buttock. Hold for a moment.

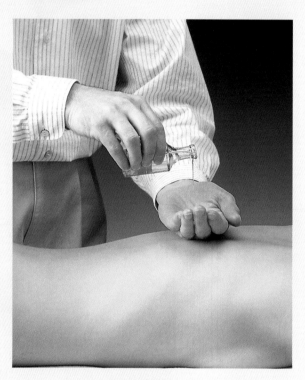

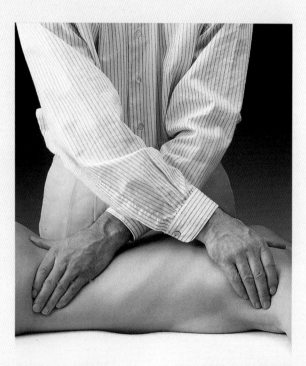

4 After a short time start to apply the massage oil. You should then take your time to make a visuall assessment of the back.

5 From the head or from the side position, effleurage your partner's back, hands on either side of the spine (not on the spine) using equal pressure throughout under your palms. Glide back up to the neck.

TIP
Ensure your partner does not get cold at this stage, as most of their body is exposed. Move up the towels, leaving the area being worked on uncovered.

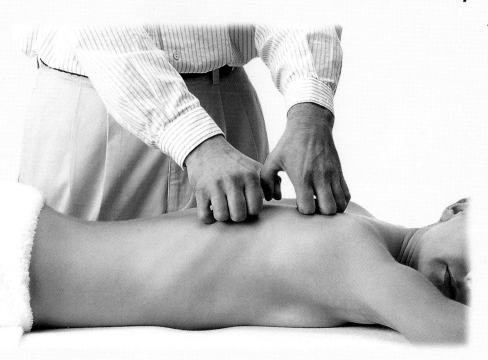

6 You can use the back of the knuckles to trace down the back, flattening the hands off at the lower back to glide back up.

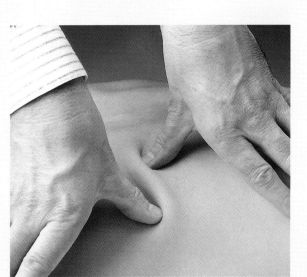

7 Use the thumb technique from the shoulder and base of the neck, downward and outward.

8 From the side, effleurage the neck gently with V of the hand, alternating kneading on neck.

9 From the head, repeat thumb pressures, pushing the muscle away on both sides of the neck and shoulders.

10 With thumbs either side of the spine, trace down the spine (lighten pressure in the sacral area). Then glide your hands back up to your partner's neck.

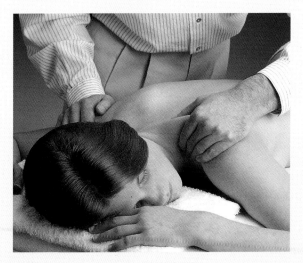

11 Muscle roll the shoulders, taking care not to pinch the skin between the fingers and thumb.

12 Working from the opposite side, knuckle or with thumbs work the rhomboid area, tracing the rib cage also. Avoid the scapula (flat of shoulder blade) and the actual spinal column.

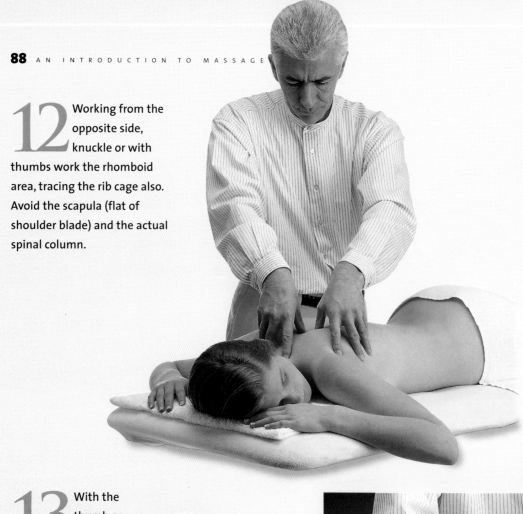

13 With the thumb or palm of the hand, trace the scapula. Knead and pick up the lateral side of muscle.

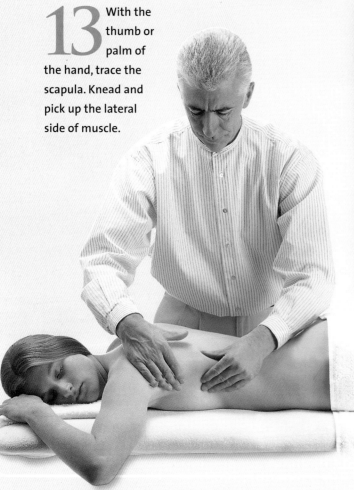

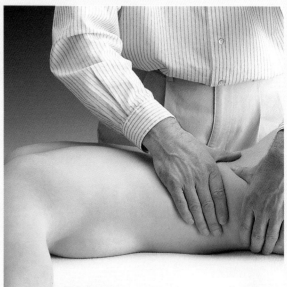

14 Apply alternate kneading to the sides of the trunk and to the gluteus at the top of the buttock.

1 Working from the other side of the body, repeat from Step 12 (see opposite).

2 From the side, apply gentle fisting in small circles from the centre of the back outward over the iliac crest to the outer gluteal (you can use tripod stance and fist one hand at a time at the opposite side). Repeat the small circles with the thumbs.

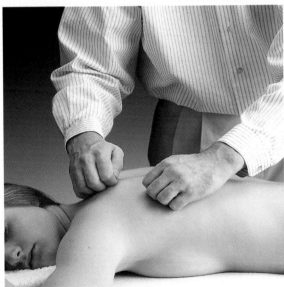

3 Repeat the fisting movement over the shoulder area.

4 Effleurage up the back from the side and glide back down.

5 Using an effleurage feathering motion, glide back up to the neck. You can move back to the head if you prefer to continue effleurage with alternate hands. Feather off to finish.

6 Cover with the towel and centre energy with one hand on the sacrum and the other hand at shoulder level. Hold the position for a moment.

7 (Optional) Add head massage by standing at the head position and gently apply fingertip rotation to the scalp with shampooing action. With very slight pulling and tugging of the hair root, run your fingers palm up through the hair to stimulate. Smooth hair down gently when finished.

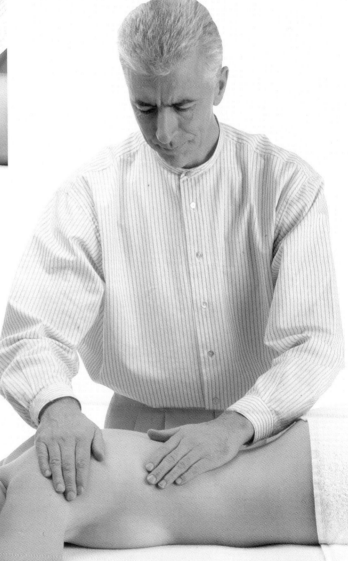

Relaxation Techniques

A successful massage will leave you stress-free and relaxed. Build on this feeling by learning relaxation techniques that you can apply anywhere at any time. If you step back from the stress and relax you will be happy and healthy and feel better equipped to cope with life's challenges.

BREATH CONTROL

Breathe in peace through your nose and breathe out tension through your open mouth. Try to visualise the word 'peace' in white large letters, and the word 'tension' in grey growing smaller with each breath.

When giving treatment, breathe with each other for three slow, deep breaths when you begin. Yogic breathing can be a great help in quieting the mind and helping you to relax. Practitioners of Hatha yoga believe that:

> *When the breath is steady,*
> *so is the mind.*

Lie comfortably and focus on your breathing. Place your hands on your abdomen and feel your breath gently flowing through your body.

MEDITATION

Meditation is a state of mind, and it is not necessary to sit in the lotus position for hours each day to achieve it. Meditation will progress with your own ability and the agility of your mind and body. To begin regular meditation practice is to take a huge step in your personal spiritual development. As well as developing the practice of stationary meditation skills, you will find moving meditations that are easy to perform. Did you know you have your own personal alarm clock? You just have to learn how to set it. Tell yourself how long you want your meditation to be before you begin and you will find with regular practice that conscious thought will step in and bring you back in your set time.

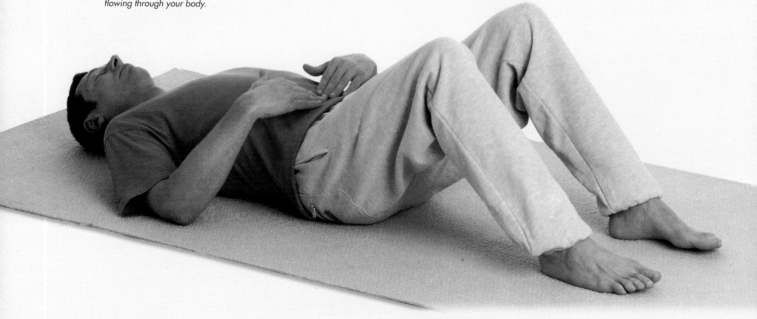

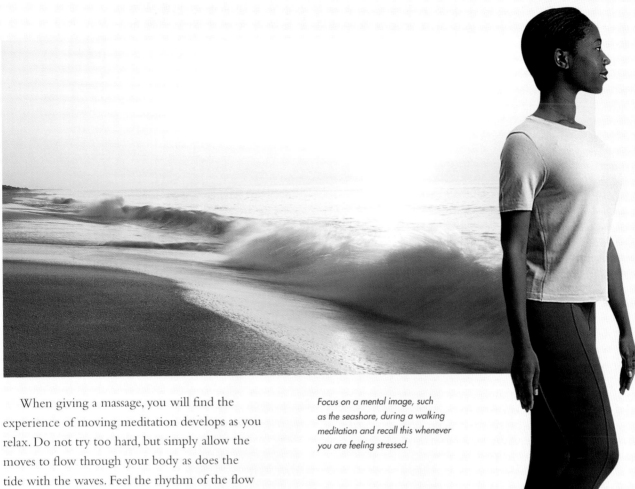

Focus on a mental image, such as the seashore, during a walking meditation and recall this whenever you are feeling stressed.

When giving a massage, you will find the experience of moving meditation develops as you relax. Do not try too hard, but simply allow the moves to flow through your body as does the tide with the waves. Feel the rhythm of the flow as you move forward and backward and from side to side, taking your momentum from the inner sounds of the beach. Initiating the idea encourages your body moves, shifting your weight, moving side to side. You will also find yourself feeling new sensations as you move your body gracefully in motion with the rhythm.

You can try this one wherever you are now. From your living room or workplace you can stand up and take a walk. Concentrate your mind on the body action of lifting your leg and placing your foot to the ground. Feel the connection with the surface beneath you. Begin to concentrate on the feel of the texture and temperature beneath your foot. Whether you are indoors or outdoors, the message receptors of your brain will help you stimulate to the sensations of connection in each part of your body now, not just your foot. Be aware of the mechanical action as you lift your limb and consciously place it down with

each step. Try this exercise again, first closing your eyes and visualising where you might like to be – in a field of long grass, on a warm, sunny, sandy beach or on a cool, stony, pebble beach. You can be taken anywhere.

This is one example of moving meditation. Try it again – you will find it difficult to plan tonight's meal and tomorrow's work schedule at the same time. You are experiencing one form of cutting out the world, enabling you to go deeper into yourself for a chosen length of time.

Transcendental Meditation is an expression of exercise for mind that seeks to induce detachment from problems and relief from anxiety. Through regular meditation, a different plane of consciousness, contemplation and relaxation can be reached.

RELAXATION: POINTERS TO GET YOU STARTED

Set the scene – warm and comfortable, with cushions, subdued lighting, and soft music.

Take the telephone off the hook or put on the answering machine to limit interruptions.

Plan how long you wish to practise meditation for – make your own appointment and make sure you keep your valuable time for yourself. By telling yourself 'I wish to meditate for a set period of time', you set your own internal alarm clock.

If you have family at home, tell them that you do not want to be disturbed during this set time.

Begin by sitting comfortably upright on the floor with a cushion under you, or in an upright chair, or lie flat on the floor, keeping your spine as straight as possible.

Close your eyes to help shut out the busy world.

Be still, calm and happy. Feel joy. Smile.

Go within and become the observer of your own thoughts, but do not engage in them – for example, the thought of shopping from the supermarket is one thing, but resist the temptation to complete your shopping mentally.

Acknowledge and appreciate any feelings or visualisation – do not hold on to them, just allow them to pass. You may experience colour, scenes, things with a symbolic meaning, or, indeed nothing at all. Do not feel cheated if you do not experience anything.

Let your thoughts slow down and become more peaceful.

You can lead your mind and body and create your own thoughts by repeating an affirmation such as 'I am a peaceful being.'

Breathe in peace and breathe out tension – visualise words entering and leaving the body.

It is wonderful and unforgettable to empty the mind and experience the state of bliss. Feel the stillness – as you are spirit, you are an integral part of the universe/cosmos – infinite.

When you open your eyes, do not rush about – enjoy tranquillity for as long as you can.

Brush yourself down; sigh with contentment.

Be thankful – feel gratitude, and smile.

You are now ready to resume your daily activities.

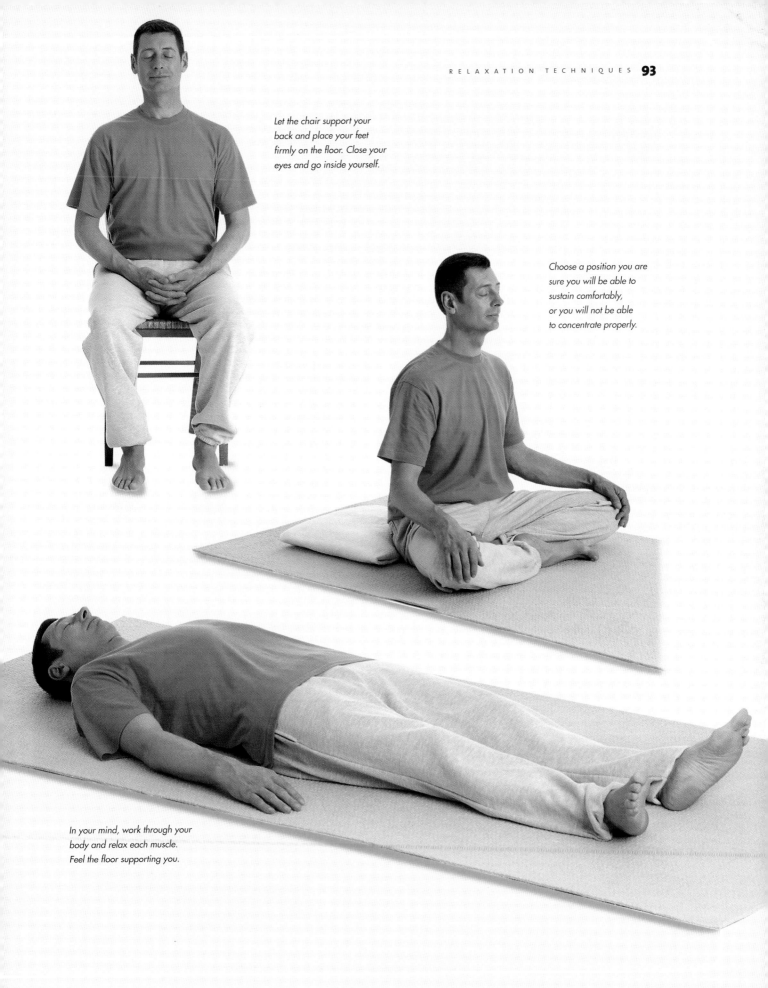

Let the chair support your back and place your feet firmly on the floor. Close your eyes and go inside yourself.

Choose a position you are sure you will be able to sustain comfortably, or you will not be able to concentrate properly.

In your mind, work through your body and relax each muscle. Feel the floor supporting you.

Visualisation

With a little imagination you can travel anywhere you like. Use photographs or create artwork to help you imagine a wonderfully relaxing world. This imaginative trip will help you to centre yourself and consequently will help you to improve your massage technique. Set aside some time for yourself, sit or lie flat, take the telephone off the hook. Close your eyes and imagine.

HOT-AIR BALLOON TRIP

Imagine you are piloting a hot-air balloon. Picture the tremendous, brightly coloured balloon. See yourself climbing into the basket. Feel the sense of wonderment as you take off. When you are airborne, see tree-tops, hills, valleys and rivers. Imagine beautiful scenery as you would like the earth to be. Look at the wonderful colours of nature. Begin the descent. Become aware of the tree-tops below you. Become aware of animals grazing in the fields. As you descend, become aware of bushes and slowly see an expanse of grass in a clearing for you to land gently. Feel stable and firm and upright. Hear the roar of the gas balloon once more as you climb over the basket, firmly placing your feet on the ground. If you feel a little unsteady, allow a loved one or someone you can trust to help you leave the balloon. Smell the grass and the flowers. Walk away from the balloon towards family or friends. Be thankful for your experience.

As an optional extension, fly above a river. The river widens into a vast lake. Absorb the deep blue-green healing tranquillity of the water. Then head to the sea. Over the ocean, feel the change in the air. Hear and see seagulls. Taste the salt on your lips. Visualise the coastline drawing nearer. Land safely, feeling rejuvenated and recharged from the trip.

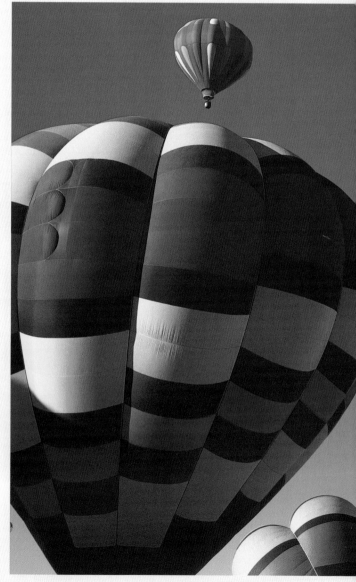

Visualisation is a technique worth mastering. If you can recall at will the feelings it engenders, you will be well equipped to face whatever challenges life throws at you.

A WALK THROUGH
A GARDEN

It does not have to be your garden, but one that your mind creates and might enjoy – a personal paradise. Go down the garden path and through a picket-fence gate. Enter fields of blooms and aromas. Visualise the blooms independently – all your favourites in abundance. Feel the spongy texture of the grass as you meander aimlessly and happily through. As you walk towards home, go back through the gate, and walk along the short gravel pathway into your room.

TAKE A TRIP TO ANOTHER PLANET

Visualise yourself getting into your own spacecraft. Pull down the hatch and you are ready to go. For peaceful meditation, wander through the galaxies and stars as you travel without gravity in awe and wonderment at the universe. For fast, invigorating travel, buckle up and hear the crowd gathered below cheer you on your way into the deep unknown. Are you brave enough to land elsewhere? Remain in your craft and bring your news home to earth to the television crews and loved ones waiting for you as you land safely. You are in control of your own destiny. You decide.

AFFIRMATIONS

Affirmations are conscious thoughts that help you direct your life as you choose. Repeating them aloud will help you to strengthen your intention and achieve your goal.

Make up an affirmation of your own that applies to your daily life. Here are some ideas to get you started – choose one that applies to you and repeat it throughout the day.

- Just for today I will not be angry. Just for today I will not worry.
- I can be what I will to be, what I choose to be.
- I am happy, loving, healthy, wealthy and whole.
- I am always in control of my own mind and body functioning.
- I will always act and react in a positive manner to any given situation.

Here is an affirmation to help you to help yourself recover from ill health:

- Every molecule, every cell, every tissue of my body constantly renews itself in perfect health. I am perfection personified.

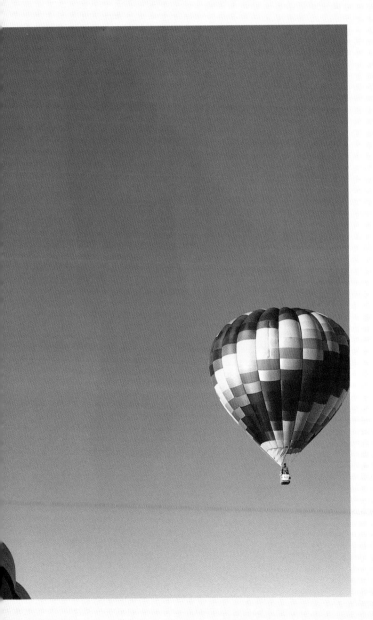

Index

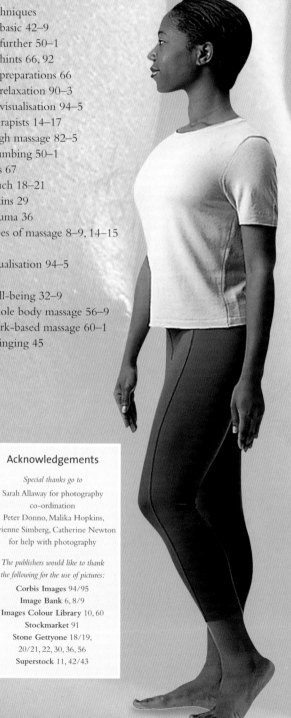

Acknowledgements

Special thanks go to
Sarah Allaway for photography
co-ordination
Peter Donno, Malika Hopkins,
Vivienne Simberg, Catherine Newton
for help with photography

*The publishers would like to thank
the following for the use of pictures:*
Corbis Images 94/95
Image Bank 6, 8/9
Images Colour Library 10, 60
Stockmarket 91
Stone Gettyone 18/19,
20/21, 22, 30, 36, 56
Superstock 11, 42/43